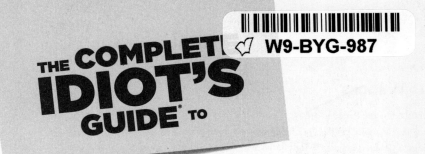

THE COMPLETE IDIOT'S GUIDE TO

Pain Relief

by Alpana Gowda, M.D., and Karen K. Brees, Ph.D.

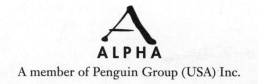

ALPHA

A member of Penguin Group (USA) Inc.

To my mother, Shail, who kissed every wound to make it feel better.
To my father, Raghava, who reached out his hand and helped me get up.
To my brother, Abhishek, who always kept me laughing.

ALPHA BOOKS

Published by the Penguin Group

Penguin Group (USA) Inc., 375 Hudson Street, New York, New York 10014, USA

Penguin Group (Canada), 90 Eglinton Avenue East, Suite 700, Toronto, Ontario M4P 2Y3, Canada (a division of Pearson Penguin Canada Inc.)

Penguin Books Ltd., 80 Strand, London WC2R 0RL, England

Penguin Ireland, 25 St. Stephen's Green, Dublin 2, Ireland (a division of Penguin Books Ltd.)

Penguin Group (Australia), 250 Camberwell Road, Camberwell, Victoria 3124, Australia (a division of Pearson Australia Group Pty. Ltd.)

Penguin Books India Pvt. Ltd., 11 Community Centre, Panchsheel Park, New Delhi—110 017, India

Penguin Group (NZ), 67 Apollo Drive, Rosedale, North Shore, Auckland 1311, New Zealand (a division of Pearson New Zealand Ltd.)

Penguin Books (South Africa) (Pty.) Ltd., 24 Sturdee Avenue, Rosebank, Johannesburg 2196, South Africa

Penguin Books Ltd., Registered Offices: 80 Strand, London WC2R 0RL, England

Copyright © 2010 by Alpana Gowda, M.D., and Karen K. Brees, Ph.D.

International Standard Book Number: 978-1-61564-017-1
Library of Congress Catalog Card Number: 2010920423

12 11 10   8 7 6 5 4 3 2 1

Interpretation of the printing code: The rightmost number of the first series of numbers is the year of the book's printing; the rightmost number of the second series of numbers is the number of the book's printing. For example, a printing code of 10-1 shows that the first printing occurred in 2010.

Printed in the United States of America

Note: This publication contains the opinions and ideas of its authors. It is intended to provide helpful and informative material on the subject matter covered. It is sold with the understanding that the authors and publisher are not engaged in rendering professional services in the book. If the reader requires personal assistance or advice, a competent professional should be consulted.

The authors and publisher specifically disclaim any responsibility for any liability, loss, or risk, personal or otherwise, which is incurred as a consequence, directly or indirectly, of the use and application of any of the contents of this book.

Most Alpha books are available at special quantity discounts for bulk purchases for sales promotions, premiums, fund-raising, or educational use. Special books, or book excerpts, can also be created to fit specific needs.

For details, write: Special Markets, Alpha Books, 375 Hudson Street, New York, NY 10014.

Publisher: *Marie Butler-Knight*

Associate Publisher: *Mike Sanders*

Senior Managing Editor: *Billy Fields*

Senior Acquisitions Editor: *Paul Dinas*

Development Editor: *Michael Thomas*

Production Editor: *Kayla Dugger*

Copy Editor: *Kelly D. Henthorne*

Cover Designer: *Kurt Owens*

Book Designers: *William Thomas, Rebecca Batchelor*

Indexer: *Tonya Heard*

Layout: *Ayanna Lacey*

Proofreader: *John Etchison*

...nts

Introduction

As a doctor, my purpose is to provide my patients with the best care possible. Each of my patients is an individual, and that means that the needs of each of my patients with pain differ. Those with acute pain must be treated differently from patients with chronic pain. For patients with chronic pain, treatment means a multidisciplinary system with the goal of restoring function and improving that patient's ability to function in everyday life.

Education is key to understanding pain and how it works in your life. In this book you'll find the information you need to become an educated consumer of health-care services.

Research has given us many new tools to manage pain more effectively. This means that if oral medications aren't providing you with relief, other options are available to you. Research continues, and every year we make significant advances in treating pain.

Pain relief is a team effort. It involves you, your physician, your surgeon, your physical therapist, and in many cases, a counselor trained to provide cognitive behavioral therapy that can help you achieve control of your pain issues.

Pain relief truly requires a multidisciplinary approach. As you read this book, you're looking for answers to your questions. How do you treat acute pain? How do you live with chronic pain? We've tried to provide helpful information that addresses your concerns.

You can't go it alone. Take advantage of the resources available to you and reach out to take the hand of those ready, willing, and able to help. Become an active participant in your own pain-relief therapies.

Use this book as a guide. Learn from it and then talk with your doctor about your concerns. Educate yourself about your medical condition. You are the person who knows you best. There is help for you, whatever your diagnosis.

How This Book Is Organized

This book is designed to be a "head to toe" primer on pain relief. From diagnosis through treatment and prevention, let this book be your guide and companion.

Part 1, Understanding Pain, tells you what pain is, how it works, and what you need to know so you're prepared to confront it head on.

Part 2, Diagnosing and Treating Pain, walks you through the various tests and procedures that can help you home in on pain.

Part 3, Pain from Head to Toe, takes you on a tour of your body, showing you how pain works in every place and what you can do about it.

Part 4, The Broader Picture of Pain, explains what happens when pain becomes an illness of its own.

Extras

This book includes four different types of sidebars to enhance your understanding of pain relief. Look for these boxes:

DEFINITION

Understanding medical language can be difficult. Here are definitions and explanations of medical terms used in this book.

POINTERS ON PAIN

Here you'll find additional important tips and information on managing pain.

STABS AND JABS

Cautions and concerns to be aware of.

SPEAKING OF PAIN

Good information on pain facts and stats.

Acknowledgments

I'd like to pay tribute to my mentors from The Ohio State University and Stanford University. My training in Physical Medicine and Rehabilitation and Pain Management has taught me to think outside the box. I am humbled by their continued interest in my learning.

Trademarks

All terms mentioned in this book that are known to be or are suspected of being trademarks or service marks have been appropriately capitalized. Alpha Books and Penguin Group (USA) Inc. cannot attest to the accuracy of this information. Use of a term in this book should not be regarded as affecting the validity of any trademark or service mark.

Understanding Pain

Pain is an unwelcome part of the human experience. Whether the result of an injury or a component of an underlying medical condition, pain makes life uncomfortable. While we all hope for a cure for pain, sometimes the best we can do is learn to manage it and reduce its impact on our daily lives.

In Part 1, we'll take an in-depth look at what pain is, how it works, and how it's measured. Everyone's experience with pain is unique, and we'll discuss how best to communicate your pain experience to your physician.

Pain Basics

In This Chapter

- Coming to terms with pain
- How pain works
- Your brain and pain
- Rethinking pain

What exactly is pain? Science has some surprising answers to that question. Beginning with the search for a definition, researchers have broadened their scope to seek clues to what causes pain, how the body and the brain recognize pain, and what happens when pain doesn't go away. In this chapter, we'll examine the cycle of pain, learn something about its underlying nature, and discuss the different approaches for treating acute and chronic pain.

Defining Pain

Before you can figure out how something works, you need to define what it is. That may seem like a simple enough task, but pain is something that can be difficult to accurately define in a few words or even in a paragraph.

Many folks have taken a stab at defining pain. One of the most widely used definitions is the one used by the International Association for the Study of Pain. They've defined pain as "an unpleasant sensory and emotional experience arising from actual or potential tissue damage or described in terms of such damage."

Another definition, preferred by the American Academy of Pain Medicine, is shorter. The Academy considers pain as "an unpleasant sensation and emotional response to that sensation."

These definitions are a start, but what exactly do they mean? Let's take a look at the first one and break it into its components.

1. The first part: "unpleasant sensory or emotional experience arising from actual or potential tissue damage." For example, actual tissue damage can result from a burn or any type of trauma. Potential tissue damage is what might happen *if* you got burned or hurt in some way. So, if you think you might get burned or injured, can you feel pain before the fact? It would appear so. Fear and worry can create pain.

2. The second part: "or described in terms of such damage." If you're not sure what that means, you're not alone.

The second definition simply condenses the first and eliminates its confusing concluding part. But is all unpleasant sensation pain? And must you get emotionally involved with the situation to feel pain?

These clinical definitions leave a great deal to be desired in terms of conveying the broad spectrum of pain, what pain means, and each person's experience with pain. Another way to look at pain is by measuring how long it lasts. By this method, we can define pain as acute or chronic.

POINTERS ON PAIN

The intensity of your pain does not always correlate with the amount of damage your body has sustained. Minor injuries may hurt a great deal, while some major injuries may not.

Acute Pain

Acute pain comes on suddenly, and often the cause of that pain can be identified quickly. In fact, that's the reason for acute pain—to get you to do something about what's causing it. It's your body's way of telling you to pay attention to what's happening and to stay out of danger.

Once you've dealt with the cause of acute pain by taking some sort of action, acute pain subsides. That's why it's called acute, as opposed to chronic pain that lingers.

Accidents are probably the main cause of acute pain, with illnesses coming in second, and surgical procedures third. It's impossible to ignore the pain of a broken bone, the pounding headache that comes with the flu, or the aftermath of surgery. After the bone has been set, you've taken medication for your flu symptoms, and your incision has healed, acute pain disappears.

It's not difficult to come up with numerous examples of acute pain. A heart attack, herniated disc, toothache, sprained ankle—the list could go on and on. But everything on the list has one thing in common: after what's causing the pain has been addressed, you're on the way to recovery … usually. But what happens when acute pain doesn't go away?

Chronic Pain

Any type of pain, whether in your back, shoulder, pelvis, or head, is considered to be chronic when it persists for three months or longer. There is some discussion among pain doctors about how long pain must linger to be called chronic. It used to be six months, but now it can be as little as one month.

 SPEAKING OF PAIN

About 9 percent of the United States population and about 18 percent of the European population suffer from chronic pain.

Chronic pain can be broken into two categories, depending upon whether the pain is affecting your nervous system (neuropathic pain) or is affecting other body tissues apart from the nerves (nociceptive pain).

It's possible to experience both neuropathic and nociceptive pain at the same time. For example, if you have a medical condition that affects your spinal column, such as spinal stenosis or a herniated disc, there can be injury to the nerves (neuropathic) and pain in surrounding muscles, tendons, and ligaments (nociceptive). In this scenario, you'll need to treat both types of pain.

Types of Pain

Pain is communication. If you're feeling pain, there is most likely a specific name for it, related to its cause. It can be helpful to become familiar with some of the most common terms for describing pain. Pain for which there is no identifiable cause is called idiopathic pain. The term doesn't imply that you're not feeling pain; it just means the doctors can't figure out what's causing it.

Phantom Limb Pain

"Pain is your body telling you that something's wrong." You've undoubtedly heard this saying numerous times. It's both true and false. It's true because that's exactly what the message is relaying. Your body is telling your brain that something is wrong with one of its parts. However, the message isn't always accurate or reliable. For example, in phantom limb pain, your brain is getting information from a body part that's no longer there.

In some cases, people who have had a limb amputated still experience pain that feels as if it's coming from that limb. This pain is called phantom limb pain, and even though the limb is gone, the pain is very real.

For many reasons, connections in the central nervous system (CNS) get mixed up, and the brain is confused. It thinks there's a signal coming from the amputated limb. That goes back to the idea that pain is in the "brain." The imprint of the lost limb is still in the brain pathway and continues to relay pain or abnormal sensations. Phantom limb pain has its own sensations and can feel like burning, squeezing, or crushing.

Anginal Pain

Anginal pain is chest pain associated with the heart and results when the blood supply to the heart muscle is disrupted. It's been described as "an elephant sitting on your chest," tightness, or a feeling of impending doom. It's not a pain that should be ignored. It's a call for immediate action.

Cancer Pain

Cancer pain may be caused by the cancer or by the means used to treat the cancer, such as chemotherapy and surgery. Treating cancer pain can be difficult. Cancer pain is challenging, as the types of pain in this broad category include everything from bone pain to nerve pain and other aches and pains, such as headaches.

Breakthrough Pain

Breakthrough pain is also called episodic pain. It's called *breakthrough* because the pain truly breaks through even when you are actively treating it and have been able to previously control it. This type of pain usually comes on very quickly but, thankfully, does not last long.

Pain Is in the Brain—and Nervous System

Your brain is just part of the story—one member of the cast that consists of your CNS and your peripheral nervous system (PNS). Your CNS is made up of your brain and your spinal cord. Your PNS is where nerves and nerve pathways are located. These two systems are connected and together they make up your entire nervous system.

Without your nervous system, you wouldn't be able to feel or acknowledge pain. That might sound like a nice idea, but it's really not. Pain is how your CNS communicates with your body to get you to take positive action to remove the cause of the pain. This is true in acute pain but not as true with chronic pain because different things are happening in the nervous system with acute pain as compared to chronic pain.

To understand how the nervous system works to communicate acute pain, let's start with an example that we're all familiar with: the paper cut. The process goes like this:

1. You pick up a piece of paper by the edge.

2. You feel a sharp sting.

3. You drop the paper and look at your finger.

4. There's a tiny cut on your finger.

5. You probably put your finger in your mouth and suck on it.

6. Your finger gradually stops hurting, and you forget all about it after several minutes.

Here's what happened:

1. The paper cut you. That's the *stimulus*.

2. Next, nerve endings in your finger felt that cut. That's the reception part of the sequence.

3. After that, those nerve endings sent a message to your spinal cord.

4. The message continued on to your brain and, like the neighborhood gossip, told it what happened. That's the transmission segment.

5. Your brain received that information and told your finger to drop the paper.

6. The brain sent hormones called endorphins to the injury site to ease the acute pain.

And that's how acute pain works.

All of that happened in a second. It's really amazing how quickly the nervous system gets the job done.

> **DEFINITION**
>
> A **stimulus** is anything that produces a response.

That's the abbreviated version of a very complicated process. Other chemical actions are also taking place after you've hurt yourself. For example, after receiving the message about your injury, your brain (in addition to telling you to drop the paper) also releases endorphins, the body's "feel good" hormones. These are responsible for reducing the intensity of the pain you feel.

At the same time, other neurochemicals that don't "feel good" are released along both the CNS and the PNS. They have other jobs to do.

The Complex Nature of Pain

Your genetic makeup has a great deal to say about how your body feels and processes pain signals. We used to think that people who faced severe pain without flinching were models of strong personal character, bravery, and a host of other positive virtues. We also tended to believe that folks who winced and flinched at minor injuries were somehow weak, crybabies, and prima donnas. As it turns out, there's much more involved than a stoic nature or a wimpy outlook on life.

You have a genetic predisposition that influences the degree to which you feel pain. Just as pain is individual, so is your genetic makeup. This means that how you process pain medications and how much pain you can tolerate are genetically influenced. So, pain can be a very different experience for different people.

Many factors can influence how much pain you feel at a given time. Your age and your sex can play a role. Scientists used to think that children didn't feel pain as intensely as adults. They now know that this is not true. Children feel pain much more intensely than do adults, for a few reasons.

Children and Pain

The most common pain that children experience is acute pain. The most common causes are injury and illness. So why do they feel pain more intensely than adults?

First of all, the neurochemicals that process pain information are developed while the fetus is in the womb. Therefore, at birth, children have the capacity to feel pain. Current research has also shown that children and infants can develop "lasting memories" of their pain experiences, which can hardwire their brains to cause problems with pain as adults.

Because children are just learning about pain, they don't know what to expect, and they can be frightened. Fear makes pain worse.

Finally, children are often undertreated for their pain. In very young children this is because they're not able to tell where it hurts or how much it hurts. This may cause them to be undertreated for their pain.

POINTERS ON PAIN

You feel pain more keenly if you're tired or under stress.

Pain and the Elderly

At the other end of the age spectrum, older adults also feel pain more intensely than their younger counterparts. This can be a result of a loss of cushioning power by cartilage breakdown in the joints and the wear and tear on them that leads to osteoarthritis. Older adults are also frequently undertreated for their pain.

Arthritis is a common condition of older people, and it can be exacerbated by the weather. Arthritis hurts more when the weather is cold and damp. Many of the elderly believe that old age and pain go together and there's not much to be done about it. If they believe that hurting is now part of life, they may not seek medical help for their pain. If they are suffering from Alzheimer's or other forms of dementia, they have the same difficulties in communicating what they are feeling as young children do.

Adults and Pain

Men and women are different! That's not news, of course, but it's an important factor in how pain is felt. Researchers have learned that when estrogen levels are high, endorphins and enkephalins (the brain's pain-fighting hormones) are also stronger and help block pain. Low estrogen levels correlate with weaker endorphins and enkephalins, and pain is felt more intensely.

This makes sense when you consider that a woman's body must prepare for the pain associated with childbirth and cope with the monthly estrogen swings of her menstrual cycle.

On the other hand, women appear to have a greater tendency than men to develop depression, which can intensify the pain experience. Depression has been linked to fluctuating hormone levels, which can result in mood swings. When these mood swings become severe enough to interfere with daily living, it's time to check in with your physician. Medication is available to help get your body back in balance.

> **SPEAKING OF PAIN**
>
> Women suffering from depression have an increased risk for fractures. With severe depression, there is a 40 percent increased risk of hip fracture over a 10-year period.

Adults who smoke experience heightened pain responses. This is partly because of decreased oxygen in the blood and partly because nicotine interrupts the normal signals of pain to the brain. People who smoke also tend to have more back pain than nonsmokers.

How Acute Pain Becomes Chronic

Generally, the longer pain persists, the greater the chance it will become chronic. Persistent pain actually can produce changes in the nervous system over time, and the brain produces proteins that it normally wouldn't. Research into this process is ongoing, and hopefully researchers will soon develop new medications that can target these proteins and stop chronic pain in its tracks.

Chronic pain doesn't respond to medication the same way acute pain does. This is why it's important to treat acute pain promptly. Doctors have learned that patients whose post-surgical pain is not treated effectively have a greater chance of that pain becoming ongoing.

In any given group of people with the same medical condition, some will develop chronic pain, and others will not. There may be a genetic component that explains why this happens. This is a current area of research.

For many years, doctors dismissed people's complaints about chronic pain as unfounded. Since there wasn't any identifiable reason for the pain to have continued, they assumed it didn't. Until research proved that chronic pain did indeed exist, it was common to blame the person for the problem. Chronic pain was thought of as psychosomatic, or "all in their heads." Unfortunately, that response did nobody any good. Today we know that chronic pain is a medical condition in its own right.

STABS AND JABS

Don't make assumptions about your pain. Coincidence isn't necessarily causation. Your doctor is the one to help you discover what's causing your pain.

Retraining the Brain

As you've read earlier in this chapter, the nervous system actually undergoes changes with chronic pain. These changes keep the signals coming, even when they no longer provide any benefit and the situation has been managed as best as possible.

Changing these signals back to more productive use takes some time and effort. This process relies on the age-old theory of mind over matter and harnesses the power of the mind-body connection. In practical terms, you can actually learn how to change the brain's activity and take an active role in your own pain relief and pain management. Some of this is done with distraction, some with re-education, and some with the power of positive thinking.

POINTERS ON PAIN

Treating chronic pain requires a multidisciplinary approach, which means combining resources from physical medicine as well as from mental health professionals.

Reconditioning the brain to change its perceptions of pain involves Cognitive Behavioral Therapy (CBT). CBT has been around a long time, and it operates from the premise that you get what you expect. This means that by changing the way you think about something, you can actually change the way you think about something. (That last sentence is not a mistake.)

CBT has problem-solving at its core. In fact, recent studies have shown that CBT can significantly alter certain areas of the brain. You can use these changes to your advantage as you work to desensitize yourself to pain.

Your physician can refer you to a licensed *psychotherapist* who will guide you through the process of learning how to retrain your brain. This is not a passive endeavor on your part, however, and you'll work one-on-one with your therapist to set goals, develop strategies, and practice new skills that will help you relieve your pain.

> **DEFINITION**
>
> A **psychotherapist** is someone with a Master's degree or a doctorate in one of the mental health disciplines who provides counseling and therapy. Psychotherapists can be psychiatrists, registered psychiatric nurses, licensed counselors, or clinical social workers.

In CBT you'll do a great deal of thinking about your pain and the ways you are currently dealing with and experiencing it. Then you'll work on learning strategies for changing those thought patterns into more positive, constructive ones. Here's an example of how CBT can work.

Suppose you have arthritis and you aren't sleeping well. In the morning you're fatigued, and this fatigue has increased the severity of your pain. You're caught in a vicious cycle. You dread going to bed because you know you're not going to sleep. You're certain that in the morning you're going to feel terrible. This is your current reality, and this is the reality you are going to change. It's a step-by-step process. Working with your therapist, you go through the following steps:

1. You identify the problem: you're not sleeping.

2. You set your goal: improved sleep and subsequent pain relief.

3. You develop strategies for meeting this goal. These strategies include:

   • Practicing sleep hygiene, which means developing a pre-bedtime routine that reduces stress and tension.

   • Checking with your physician to see whether your pain medications may be responsible for your insomnia. Sometimes just changing the time of day you take them is all you need to do to improve the quality of your sleep.

   • Re-envisioning bedtime as a peaceful, relaxing end of the day and a restorative part of your pain-relief therapy.

   • Discussing relaxation techniques, such as biofeedback and self-hypnosis, with your therapist and incorporating these into your end-of-day routine.

You know that your arthritis is not going to be cured, but you also know that your attitude affects how you feel. By changing this one attitude toward sleep, you've begun to retrain your brain to now see sleep as attainable, and you no longer dread the bed.

Here's one more example of how CBT can help when you're faced with chronic pain. Feeling powerless over your pain makes each day seem like a series of insurmountable hurdles. It's a constant uphill struggle.

If you have *fibromyalgia*, you understand all too well what that feels like. You may find yourself at one of two extremes: in the first case, you're in denial. You're determined to live life just as you did before fibromyalgia and you're constantly frustrated that you can't. In the second case, you're convinced nothing you can do will ever get you back in control of your life. Both extremes have a great deal in common, and both can benefit from CBT.

DEFINITION

Fibromyalgia is a syndrome with symptoms that include fatigue and pain in soft tissues, along with areas of extreme tenderness (called tender points).

The first step is accepting the reality of the situation: you have fibromyalgia. The second step is figuring out how to live with it—not deny that it's there, but make some adjustments to improve the quality of your life.

Overdoing it can be just as self-defeating as not doing anything. The key is pacing yourself. Working with your therapist, you learn how to set priorities and develop coping skills that will help you get through the day without trying to do everything. You also get some practice in saying one simple word: "No."

Learning your limitations isn't giving up. Accepting your medical diagnosis isn't giving in. Just as with the person dealing with arthritis, your pain won't disappear, but you'll be able to manage it and not let it control your life.

Goals for Treating Acute and Chronic Pain

The goal for treating acute pain is simple and straightforward: find the source of the pain and treat it. The focus is on correcting the injury that has caused the pain, performing the surgery or dressing the wound, and making the person as comfortable as possible during the healing process that follows. In addition to treating the cause, treating the symptoms provides pain relief while the injury heals.

Treating chronic pain, however, requires a different approach. The goal then becomes one of increasing the person's ability to function so the person can go about his or her daily routine.

Sometimes the reason for chronic pain can't be found. In that case, treating chronic pain requires a multidisciplinary approach. This may entail psychological counseling, physical and occupational rehabilitation, and ongoing emotional support. Combining different therapies can be helpful in addressing chronic pain. These therapies can include the following:

- Medications
- Cognitive Behavioral Therapy
- Physical therapy
- Interventional therapy

Learning to live with pain is challenging. You may not be able to live pain-free, but with a combined therapeutic approach, you can learn to manage pain and return to a more normal life.

The Least You Need to Know

- Pain can be broken into two types: acute and chronic.
- Your perceptions of pain are in large part genetically based.
- Acute pain will go away after the cause has been treated.
- When the cause of chronic pain is not found, the goal becomes one of learning to manage it rather than to cure it.
- Cognitive Behavioral Therapy can help empower you to live with pain on your own terms.

The Subjective Nature of Pain

In This Chapter

- Personal aspects of pain
- Evaluating pain in infants and children
- Pain intensity scales
- Pain's ripple effects

"I feel your pain." Actually, you can't. You can feel sympathy for the person who is experiencing pain, but you can't share the experience. Your early experiences with pain define pain for you, and your experiences are uniquely your own.

Your Point of View

Your frame of reference is your point of view. It's the way you interpret events around you, and you begin developing it in early childhood. Your point of view is schooled by your experiences. For example, if someone receives an award, you think how you would feel and project those feelings onto that person.

The same holds true for a less pleasant situation. If someone is in an accident and suffers an injury, you think how you would feel in similar circumstances and expect the person involved feels the same way you would.

To make matters more complex, if you're a person with a high *pain threshold*, you may come across to others as callous and uncaring. If you have a low threshold for pain, you may be seen as someone who exaggerates a situation and makes a mountain out of a molehill.

DEFINITION

Your **pain threshold** is the point where you become aware of feeling pain. It's different from your pain tolerance level, which is the amount of pain you can stand.

Using ourselves and our own experiences as a frame of reference is the best we can do, however. It's all part of being human. Sometimes we come fairly close to what others are experiencing, and other times we miss the mark entirely. Why is this so? The explanation is that pain is personal, and we all experience it differently. One person's minor twinge may feel excruciating to someone else. And both people are correct.

As you can see, this can make describing your pain to someone else, including your doctor, quite a challenge. In addition, other factors have a bearing on how you feel pain from day to day, so even with yourself, describing pain is never easy.

Regardless of how you're feeling inside, the face you show in public may be quite different from how you react in the privacy of your home. Some cultures and ethnic groups view tears as a sign of weakness and complaining as evidence of a lack of moral fiber, while other cultures and ethnic groups have no such constraints, and emotional expression running the gamut from tears to wailing is encouraged.

While individuals from both cultures experience pain, the way they express that pain is conditioned by their upbringing. This can make diagnosis difficult for both the person in pain as well as the health-care provider, especially when the patient and the health-care provider come from different cultural backgrounds.

Age Matters

As a general rule, children are more likely to encounter acute pain, and adults tend to deal with more chronic pain. However, this general rule, like all rules, seems to have been made to be broken. At both ends of the spectrum of life, communicating how one feels and conveying important information about pain can be difficult.

Infants

To a disinterested party, all babies' crying sounds the same. To a parent, however, each cry means something different, and it doesn't take a new parent long to learn what her infant is trying to tell her with each cry. Hunger, fatigue, boredom, and pain all have a different sound. They also have different facial expressions.

For infants, pain is diffused throughout the body. The face is still a good indicator of an infant's pain. Signs include:

- Closed eyes and furrowed brow, with eyelids close together
- Nose flattened out
- Tongue cupped
- Mouth tense and open in a rectangular form

In addition, infants feeling acute pain will display more shallow and rapid breathing and an increased pulse rate. Their skin will redden noticeably as they cry, although an infant whose color is overly pale may be in acute pain or shock.

Chronic pain in infants can be more difficult to determine. Infants experiencing chronic pain may not show the same signs as they would with acute pain. Sometimes they become lethargic and nonresponsive.

Older infants may thrash around, hold a limb still, or roll their heads from side to side. Whatever your child is doing that is out of the ordinary is a clue, and it's your cue to call the doctor.

As a parent, trust your instincts. If you think your infant is in pain, you are probably right. Infants in pain cannot usually be consoled by simply rocking or nursing. Always check with your child's pediatrician if you have any questions or concerns.

Infants used to not receive any anesthetics for routine medical procedures such as circumcision because it was believed they did not feel pain the same way older children or adults do. We now know this is not true, and in fact, infants can feel pain *more* acutely.

Do not accept anyone telling you that your child will "get over it" or that "she won't feel it." These statements are false. Infants can safely be given local anesthetics to numb an area that must be treated. In fact, we now know that the more we do to relieve infants' pain early on, the greater their ability to not have "lasting memory" of the pain, which could affect the way they perceive and deal with pain as adults.

Children

Children and accidents seem to go together, and childhood is liberally sprinkled with a substantial amount of scrapes and sprains, cuts, and broken bones. For children, after the cuts have been washed and dressed or the broken bones set, healing begins. Medications can ease the pain.

Childhood is also the time when we learn lifetime habits for dealing with pain. Peer pressure and parental reactions are the key elements in determining how a child negotiates this learning process.

For example, if every bump and bruise is treated as a major event, your child will see it this way as well and will experience more pain. The opposite is also true. If you take the minor scrapes in stride, your child will, too, and will tend to see them as not overly painful. So the same minor injury may be reported by two different children at different ends of the pain scale.

For more serious pain issues in young children, if the pain is internal and a symptom of illness, diagnosis and treatment can be more challenging.

Infants and toddlers can't tell you where or how much it hurts, and often their pain is undertreated. This is where a parent's intuitive sense is invaluable in helping the doctor arrive at a diagnosis so treatment and pain relief can begin. Parents know when their child is hurting and when changes in behavior warrant a trip to the doctor. It's important to follow your instincts here and become your child's advocate.

"Where does it hurt?" is the parent's usual question to an older child. Older children can tell you where it hurts and can use a pain scale to help you find out what they are experiencing (see "Putting a Number on Pain" later in this chapter).

Adults

For many adults, pain (both feeling it and doing something about it) is a matter of priorities. Stereotypes of men gritting their teeth in the face of horrible pain and of women swooning at the sight of someone in pain have played fast and loose with the facts. To some extent, cultural expectations determine our reactions to pain, both ours and pain being experienced by someone else.

Women tend to report that they experience pain more frequently and more severely than do men. Women also tend to seek treatment for pain early on, whereas men frequently postpone this treatment.

There are some differences in how men and women experience pain. Some of these differences can be traced to hormones. Some pain is unique to women (menstrual pain and childbirth pain), and some is unique to men (testicular pain and pain associated with inflammation of the prostate gland).

Women are more apt to experience pain from the following:

- Migraine headaches (see Chapter 10)

- Fibromyalgia (see Chapter 20)

- Cystitis (see Chapter 17)

- Temporomandibular joint problems (see Chapter 10)

- Lupus

- Rheumatoid arthritis (see Chapter 20)

- Complex regional pain syndrome (see Chapter 19)

POINTERS ON PAIN

During the menstrual cycle, women tend to report experiencing greater sensitivity to pain.

Men are more apt to experience pain due to the following:

- Musculoskeletal injuries

- Cluster headaches (see Chapter 10)

- Pancreatitis (see Chapter 17)

- Gallbladder (see Chapter 17)

Regardless of the medical conditions contributing to chronic pain or the external circumstances leading to acute pain, the ways in which men and women respond to that pain are generally a result of conditioning from childhood.

Acute pain tends to occur with the same frequency throughout our life spans, but chronic pain is more common in adults than in children. Chronic pain is not a normal part of aging, however, and is a condition that can be treated. Often, adults think that pain is just part of growing older, and they've given up trying to find relief.

SPEAKING OF PAIN

Statistics compiled by the Centers for Disease Control (CDC) report that 25 percent of adults in the United States experienced pain in the previous month, and for 10 percent of these people, the pain lasted a year or longer.

Older adults tend to move more slowly, and childhood's skinned knees are replaced by the aches and pains associated with wear and tear, such as those symptomatic of osteoarthritis. Sometimes, however, acute pain visits the elderly as well. Falls and accidents are serious situations with older adults.

Bones may have become brittle with osteoarthritis, and footing can become unsteady, as balance is compromised by age. Unfortunately, falls among the elderly frequently result in fractured hips, which can be life-threatening.

If you are a relative of an older adult with dementia, you may need to become an advocate for that person, especially if that person is in a care facility. In some cases, these individuals are undertreated for pain, but they deserve the same consideration as everyone else. Some of the same principles used in assessing pain with children apply here, such as pictorial pain scales (see "Wong-Baker Faces" later in this chapter).

Stress and Fatigue

Both stress and fatigue can make the pain experience worse. When you experience pain, you become tense. That tension makes the pain worse, and you feel stressed, which also makes the pain worse. If your pain persists, you can reach a point where you feel nothing but the pain. This increases your stress and adds to your fatigue. It's truly a vicious cycle. Managing stress and relieving fatigue are key to decreasing the severity of how you experience pain.

Stress is neither good nor bad. It's how we react to a *stressor* in our environment that affects how severe our pain is. In the short term, the body releases hormones that prepare you to either flee or fight when faced with a stressful situation. For this brief period, feelings of pain are suppressed. If the stress continues, however, those hormones get used up, and the pain returns to full strength.

DEFINITION

A **stressor** is any kind of stimulus that activates your body's stress response. It can be short term or chronic.

When your nerves are "on edge," you're going to have a heightened pain experience. Likewise with fatigue. Pain can rob you of restful sleep, leaving you fatigued the next day. Without proper rest, pain feels worse. You can't sleep, but you're exhausted. Eventually, you reach your limit, and the pain seems unbearable.

Personality and Pain

Does your personality determine to what extent you'll feel pain? We do know that people with high levels of anxiety have high perceptions of pain. But what about the optimists and the pessimists among us?

"This isn't going to hurt a bit." You've heard that line countless times. Turns out it's pretty good psychology. Our perceptions of pain are influenced by our expectations of pain. If we believe something is going to be painful, we tense up, anticipating the worst. However, if we believe something, such as an injection, isn't going to be more than a pinprick, we relax and the procedure is over with before we know it.

The person in that first scenario is going to feel more pain than the person in the second one. It's the mind-body connection at work. Your brain actually tells your body what's going to happen, and the body responds accordingly. Of course this doesn't work in extreme conditions, but for minor medical procedures or daily coping with aches and pains, it's good information to know. Put on your best face, and you'll actually feel better.

Putting a Number on Pain

Even though our perceptions of pain are personal, sometimes it's important that others get a fairly accurate idea of what we're experiencing. This applies especially to medical care providers who need to know what to do to help us.

Several different pain intensity scales have been devised to help providers try to do just that. Some are useful for children and adults who are trying to communicate through a language barrier. Some are used by nurses and other critical care personnel to assess the pain levels of hospitalized patients who are unable to communicate orally.

A great deal of diagnostic information in medicine is gathered through reviewing your medical history and medical testing, such as that provided by blood work and imaging tests. Numbers tell the story in these tests, and fitting your results into the range that's considered normal isn't difficult to do.

If your blood sugar comes in at a reading of 104, and the normal range of values is 1 to 100, you can tell at a glance that your level is a bit high. If your combined cholesterol is 267, you can look at your lab report and see that the number to shoot for is under 200. You know then, in both of these examples, exactly where you stand. The next step is to do something to correct the situation.

When it comes to diagnosing the level of pain you're experiencing, however, these tests are woefully inadequate. There's no normal range of values for pain, and only you can explain what you are feeling. Still, some tools can help you put a number, or at least a face, on your pain. These tools are called pain intensity scales, and they're useful for everyone—children, the elderly, the developmentally disabled, and the memory-impaired. Some are entirely visual, some are numerical, and some are in questionnaire form.

Pain intensity scales can be used to give a benchmark figure, and later in the course of your treatment, they're helpful as a comparison tool to see how well you're doing. Here are some of the more common ones you're likely to encounter.

Verbal Rating Scale

This is the simplest of the scales. You are asked to rate your pain as none, mild, moderate, or severe. One drawback is that you need to be verbal. Another drawback is that this scale doesn't have any way to account for pain that fluctuates in intensity at different times or under different circumstances. The benefit is that it's a quick assessment of a specific moment in time.

Visual Analogue Scales

This scale is a simple horizontal line. At one end it's marked "no pain," and at the other end it's marked "worst pain." You use a pencil to make an X or some other mark at some point along the scale that more or less corresponds to the pain you are experiencing. As with the verbal rating scale, this one doesn't help you explain fluctuations in your pain level, but you don't have to be verbal to make your "X."

Numeric Rating Scale

This scale goes back to the numbers to try to get a fix on your pain. It's one step more sophisticated than the verbal rating scale. It ranges from 0 to 10, with 0 being no pain and 10 being severe pain. Like the visual analogue scale, it's a horizontal line. Unlike the other scales, this one has several steps to complete. The line is broken into three segments. Each segment has three levels. At the beginning is a 0 for "no pain." From there:

- 1–3 (mild pain)
- 4–6 (moderate pain)
- 7–10 (severe pain)

First you are asked to give a number to the pain you are feeling at that moment. If it's mild but a bit bothersome, you might mark a "2."

Then you're asked to assign a number to your pain when it's at its worst. You remember that it kept you awake last night, so you might decide to mark a "7."

Next you're asked to assign a number to your pain when it's at its least. This might rate a "1."

Finally, you're asked at what number the pain is acceptable for you. If you're like most of us, you'd be tempted to mark "0," but you realize that having no pain at all may not be possible. No pain is the best outcome, but sometimes it's not realistic, so you may decide to mark "2."

POINTERS ON PAIN

The real value of pain intensity scales is in comparing your ratings over time. If your rating next week is higher than it was this week, that says your pain perception has changed. If it's lower, your pain management program may be working.

Wong-Baker Faces

This instrument was created to help children over the age of three (and adults as well) put a face to their pain. It's frequently used in hospitals and other clinical settings to get a baseline of pain prior to treatment. The six faces represent expressions from happy through neutral to very sad. You're asked to simply point to the face that best expresses what you are feeling.

The advantage of this scale is that it can be used if you aren't able to verbally communicate. The drawback is its very general, basic nature.

STABS AND JABS

Be honest! Do your best to give an accurate reading of your pain without minimizing or exaggerating it.

A Better Measure of Pain

Verbal and numeric pain measurement scales have their purposes, and they can be helpful for health-care personnel in addressing acute pain. For chronic pain, however, you need something more than lines on paper or numbers checked off in a box.

The real measure of chronic pain is looking at how you can function with pain. That's the litmus test. If someone has difficulty walking before treatment and is able to walk more easily with less pain after treatment, that's a better indicator of pain level than the number she gave to rate her pain.

If sitting causes you pain in your hip, and you receive anti-inflammatory medications that permit you to sit without pain, your improved function is a good indicator of your pain level.

Understanding Pain's Impact

Pain can be more than a signal that something is amiss with your body. It has far-reaching implications for your life that you may not have considered. Knowing how pain may affect how you live your life can empower you to make positive changes and minimize its negative impact. Understanding pain will also decrease fear and anxiety. As science now tells us, decreasing anxiety has a large impact on also decreasing pain.

Pain and Depression

Chronic pain and depression have a bit of a circular relationship. Depression can create physical symptoms, including pain, and chronic pain can lead to depression. In plain terms, physical pain can create psychological pain that can have wide-ranging effects on your life, relationships, career, and family. Breaking free of this cycle is essential to your physical and mental well-being.

Depression is a treatable medical condition. It's not "all in your head," and you can't just "snap out of it." The mind-body connection is a very powerful one, and there is a specific physiology of depression.

Certain medical conditions, such as Parkinson's disease, thyroid disease, and cancer, have depression as one of their symptoms, along with pain. Coronary artery disease and depression also have a strong connection. Certain medications used to treat various pain conditions can produce depression as a side effect.

POINTERS ON PAIN

Studies have linked depression with coronary artery disease. One study found that people with depression who had a heart attack were four times more likely to die within six months than those who were not depressed. Bottom line: treat your depression for life.

Depression intensifies pain, and pain intensifies depression. The situation becomes more and more stressful, and stress intensifies both depression and pain. See your doctor and discuss treatment if you have any of the following symptoms:

- Feeling blue or down for two weeks or longer
- Insomnia and other changes in sleep habits
- Weight gain or loss that hasn't been planned
- Difficulty concentrating
- Feelings that life isn't worth the trouble
- Thoughts of suicide
- Loss of interest in activities that used to give you pleasure
- Loss of energy

If you see any of these symptoms in yourself, have a talk with your doctor. If you are suffering from depression, treatment is available. Treating depression can work wonders in giving you pain relief.

Pain and Sleep

The less sleep you have, the greater pain you have. Your body needs rest to heal and to stock up on energy to face the new day. When pain keeps you awake, you deplete your energy stores, and you can't fight pain if you're running on empty.

The symptoms of a sleep disorder have much in common with the symptoms of depression. You can't concentrate, you're irritable, and you're exhausted. Sometimes it's the pain that's keeping you awake. For example, patients with fibromyalgia often exhibit disturbed sleep patterns, which raises havoc with their rest (see Chapter 20).

Sometimes sleeplessness is a side effect of your medications. Check with your pharmacist or your physician to see whether this is the case. Many medications are available for treating pain, and changing your meds may make a world of difference in how you sleep.

More and more research is also telling us that lack of sleep can cause certain neurochemicals to be released, and these neurochemicals can actually increase your pain.

POINTERS ON PAIN

Develop a pre-bedtime routine that supports relaxation: quiet reading, a warm bath, a light snack, and a regular time for turning out the lights. Avoid conflict, exercise, caffeine, and alcohol.

Sleep studies are available to help pinpoint what's wrong, if changing your pre-bedtime habits doesn't improve your sleep. Your physician can refer you to a sleep study clinic.

Pain and Sexuality

Decreased energy and increased pain do not make for a romantic evening. Sometimes the decreased libido is the result of your medication. For example, use of opioids for prolonged periods of time can decrease testosterone levels in both men and women, and low testosterone can dampen desire.

Check with your doctor about a possible change in medication and get your love life back on track.

Pain can make movement difficult, but learning how to move without intensifying the pain can make your sex life enjoyable once again. The Arthritis Foundation has a free, helpful booklet, "Guide to Intimacy," which gives good information on how to restore this important part of your life to its rightful place. Check Appendix B in the back of this book for contact information.

Counseling can also help. Cognitive Behavioral Therapy, which helps you understand why you feel the way you do and gives you skills for coping with pain, works very well for patients with chronic pain to help make positive changes in the bedroom.

Pain and the Workplace

Even if not suffering from a work-related injury, many people in the workplace are coping with chronic pain. Simple ergonomic changes at the desk can make the workplace amicable. Ask your human resources representative for assistance.

> ☞ **SPEAKING OF PAIN**
>
> According to an Ortho-McNeil's survey, between 1996 and 2006, there was a 38 percent increase in chronic pain among the entire U.S. full-time workforce.

Tips for coping with pain on the job include the following:

- Taking breaks as you need them
- Changing positions frequently
- Joining a workplace wellness program
- Using an ergonomic mouse, keyboard, and chair

If you need more information on how to modify your work environment, check out the Job Accommodation Network (JAN), a free service of the Office of Disability Employment Policy (ODEP) of the U.S. Department of Labor.

JAN can give you all kinds of help regarding accommodations for the workplace. Their website is www.jan.wvu.edu.

Pain and Family Issues

Pain changes the family dynamic. It is difficult for families to accept seeing their loved ones live with chronic pain, but the pendulum swings both ways. If you're struggling with pain issues, you may feel resentment toward your family members who are pain-free. You may feel anger and helplessness.

Some folks coddle their loved ones and become overprotective, and others have a hard time even acknowledging the pain. Family counseling can be a great help in re-establishing a healthy family dynamic. A mental health professional can help you learn how to relieve stress and make your family stronger.

Pain will occupy as much of your life as you let it. You can't keep it away from you or from a loved one, but you can learn ways to manage it and keep it from controlling your life.

The Least You Need to Know

- Your childhood experiences with pain determine how you'll react to pain as an adult.
- Pain intensity scales can help you establish a benchmark for pain.
- Trust your instincts as a parent, when you feel your child is in pain. Pain should be treated in children.
- Depression, lack of sleep, and fatigue can make chronic pain worse. Treating these conditions can help relieve your pain.

Diagnosing and Treating Pain

Sometimes you know the reason for your pain, but other times you may need to seek medical advice for diagnosis and treatment. Whether your pain is the result of an injury or a symptom of an underlying medical condition, you have options. Whatever the cause of your pain, there is help available for you.

Working With Your Doctor

In This Chapter

- Meeting your pain specialist
- Gathering essential information
- Keeping important records
- Developing a treatment plan

In your quest for pain relief, your primary health-care provider is the place to start. If you've had regular physical examinations, your physician already knows a good deal about your health. Now that you're faced with pain issues, your doctor will be able to recommend a course of treatment or refer you to a pain specialist. Often, a multidisciplinary approach to pain relief, one that includes many health-care professionals, produces the most satisfactory results.

Who Are Pain Specialists?

In this modern age, medicine has become defined by specialty practices. As research provides us with more and more information and more possibilities for diagnosis and treatment, the multidisciplinary approach has supplemented the general practice physician and provided more resources to help manage pain more efficiently. Your team to help you gain control of your pain may include doctors, physical therapists, occupational therapists, psychologists, acupuncturists, chiropractors, and more.

Pain physicians are doctors who provide individualized diagnostic and treatment plans for people with chronic pain issues. These physicians devote their careers to studying and treating pain. They research what causes pain, what makes it worse, what makes it better, how pain changes the body's responses to stimuli, and what techniques can be used to provide relief.

A physician who is a pain specialist may come from any of the numerous fields of medicine, including anesthesiology, physical medicine and rehabilitation (*physiatry*), neurology, and psychiatry.

DEFINITION

Physiatry is the field of physical medicine and rehabilitation. Physiatrists are also called PM&R physicians for short. These physicians are nerve, muscle, and bone experts who treat a wide array of conditions, ranging from sports injuries to strokes, spinal cord injuries, and brain injuries.

Pain specialists are generally certified in pain management by the board of a particular specialty practice; for example, the American Board of Physical Medicine and Rehabilitation, the American Board of Psychiatry and Neurology, or the American Board of Anesthesiology.

Another avenue of certification is to become board certified in pain medicine through the American Board of Pain Medicine. After completing the requirements, the physician becomes a diplomate (someone holding a diploma) of the American Board of Pain Medicine.

Many specialty practices fall under the umbrella of pain medicine, and your physician may specialize in any of them. Some specialty practices include the following:

- Sports injuries
- Back and neck pain
- Cancer pain
- Pelvic pain
- Complex regional pain syndrome
- Headache
- Fibromyalgia
- Orofacial pain

Your physician is also likely to belong to a specific professional association, such as the American Academy of Pain Management, the American Pain Society, or the American Academy of Pain Medicine.

☞ **SPEAKING OF PAIN**

Pain specialists may practice within a hospital setting, clinic, or private practice.

What to Expect at Your First Appointment

After your consultation with your primary health-care provider, you may be referred to a pain specialist. Your primary care provider may also try some physical therapy and medications to help you before referring you to the specialist. Often, if you respond to this treatment and are comfortable working with your primary care doctor, this treatment will work out fine.

If you have been referred to a pain specialist, your medical records will be sent on ahead of your first appointment. It's a good idea to call a day or two before that first appointment to be sure your records have arrived. If they haven't, that extra time will permit you to check up on their progress and ensure the records are there when you are.

The alternative is to request a copy of your records and have them with you at the time of initial evaluation. Remember to request any notes that your doctor took about your pain complaints, operation records relating to your current pain (this includes injection records), and diagnostic testing reports and films from your pain specialist. This step will save both you and the pain specialist much time.

This is also the time to sit down at the computer or with pen and paper and outline all the questions and concerns you have. Spend some time thinking about these issues and keep your list where you can add to it as new thoughts occur. Finally, when you're satisfied you've got everything listed, organize your list by grouping similar items together.

For example, you may have questions about the pain specialist's training and area of specialty practice. You may also want to know how many cases similar to yours the pain specialist treats on an annual basis. These questions will be grouped together. Another group of questions may concern your symptoms, and still another section may involve questions about possible treatments.

After you've gotten your list organized, place it in your medical file folder. If you don't have a personal medical file, it's time to compile one. Include all your surgeries (with dates), past illnesses, and the names and dosages of whatever medications you're currently taking. This is critical information for your pain doctor. A personal medical file saves time at the doctor's office, and you won't overlook anything because you feel rushed.

If you've had any recent x-rays or films done of the area that is bothering you, you may not only want to bring along the report but the actual hard copy of the study. Many physicians would like to see the actual films to get a clear visual picture of the area of concern. You may want to go to the hospital or clinic where you got those films taken and ask them to lend you the films and give you a copy of the report before your appointment with your pain doctor.

POINTERS ON PAIN

These are your medical documents; you can choose to hang on to them for future use and to show them to other doctors. The hospital or imaging center, however, may charge a fee for providing you with these documents.

Your First Appointment

You'll be asked to arrive up to an hour before your scheduled appointment with the doctor. Although it is difficult to arrive this early, most pain physicians have extensive paperwork that they need to fill out to help them understand all your pain complaints. This paperwork is often added to your medical records and read over thoroughly by your pain specialist. Sometimes you can request this paperwork to be mailed to your home prior to the appointment so you can fill it out at your leisure. Ask your doctor if this is an option.

During this time you'll fill out all the necessary forms, and the staff will enter everything into the computer. You'll need to bring a picture ID with you to that first appointment. Because of new federal privacy regulations, information cannot be divulged to third parties without your consent, and your doctor needs visual proof of your identity before treating you.

Take your insurance card with you. The receptionist who checks you in will ask for your ID and your insurance card so she can make copies for their records. The originals will be returned to you.

POINTERS ON PAIN

When filling out the questionnaire, don't forget to list any dietary supplements and herbal preparations you have been taking. Many of these have side effects that may be involved in your symptoms.

Next you'll fill out a questionnaire that seeks information about your medical history, your symptoms, and your concerns. This is where your personal medical file will be a lifesaver. If you've got everything listed, it will be a cinch to transfer the information to the form. If you've made a copy, ask whether you can simply attach this to the doctor's form.

Among the papers will be one that discusses privacy issues. You'll sign a paper that says you understand your privacy rights and that you give the doctor permission to treat you and to request copies of your medical records from places where you have received prior treatment. This paper is required by the Health Insurance Portability and Accountability Act (HIPAA) of 1996.

Meeting the Doctor

Finally, you're ready to meet the doctor. You'll have an initial conversation during which you'll discuss the reason or reasons for your visit and the doctor will go over all the items you've checked on the questionnaire. This is the time for you to ask the questions you have prepared ahead of time. If you don't understand the answers, say so. Sometimes doctors speak a medical language that is confusing to the layperson. Just let the doctor know when this happens, and she'll use language that's easier for you to understand.

POINTERS ON PAIN

Take someone with you for the first appointment with a new doctor. You'll be stressed, and that person can write down the answers to your questions so you don't have to worry that you'll forget what you've been told.

The doctor needs to hear from you directly, so if you bring someone with you, be sure to advise your companion that her role is strictly as recorder. It is always a good idea to have moral support, but only you know how you feel, even if you can't express it as well as you would like.

After your conversation, the doctor will conduct a physical examination that probably will include sending you to have specific diagnostic imaging tests. Even though you're anxious to get started on your treatment, you'll need to be patient and not expect everything to fall into place at this first visit. The test results will need to be evaluated. After the evaluation has been completed, you'll return to the doctor for a discussion of the findings. Prior to this next appointment, the doctor will probably ask you to start keeping a pain profile.

You may or may not leave the pain doctor's office on the first visit with a prescription for new medications. It all depends upon your specific pain issues and your pain doctor's treatment policy. Sometimes physicians will be able to prescribe medications or treatments after the initial meeting, while at other times this may not be possible until they have had time to formulate a plan specifically tailored for you. Unfortunately, if you have had chronic pain—pain that has lasted at least several months—the doctor will need to see you a few times to chart the right course of action for you.

Keeping a Pain Profile

Before your doctor can prescribe a course of treatment, she'll need specific information so the treatment will have the best possible chance of a positive outcome. If you're not familiar with a pain profile, it's similar to a journal or a daily log in which you keep track of what you feel, when you feel it, how it feels, and what you do about it.

You know that pain is a highly individualized experience and that the way you feel pain is unique to you. That's really all that matters—your perceptions of your pain. The first order of business is to develop a list of terms that refer to pain and decide how you will define them for yourself. For some people, a throb is less intense than an ache, but for others, the opposite is true. You'll have to decide for yourself how to use these terms.

For example, if you wake up in the morning and your knee hurts, you'll decide whether that hurt is an ache, a throb, a stab, a burn, a tingle, or something else. You identify the type of pain. Whenever you feel that particular type of pain again, you'll refer to it in the same way. Don't call it an ache one day and a throb the next, for example, if it's the same type of pain.

Next, you put a value on that pain. Imagine feeling no pain at all. You would give that a value of 0. Then think about the worst possible pain you can imagine. You would give that pain a value of 10. With those parameters in place, you can now give that hurting knee a value. Let's say you decide it's a 5. It's troublesome, you can't forget about it, but you're not writhing in agony on the floor either.

You enter this information into your pain profile. You can organize your profile into columns, paragraphs, or whatever works for you. It just needs to be consistent in form, constantly updated, and easy to read. Here's one example of how a page might look:

Date and Time	6/26/10 7:00 A.M.
Symptom	Woke up with knee throbbing.
Pain Level	5
Action	Took 2 Tylenol.

After you've been up and around for a while, suppose the pain gets better. You decide it's now a 2. You record this in your pain profile.

Time	8:00 A.M.
Pain Level	2

Or, conversely, it's getting worse with every movement, and now it's definitely a 7. You add this information to your pain profile. Either way, you've established a baseline and charted where your pain is going.

As you go through your day, keep track of what you're feeling, how you're feeling, and what you're doing when you notice the pain. It might be that exercise improves your symptoms, or the opposite may hold true—rest is the only thing that seems to help.

What are you doing for your pain? Do you take a nonsteroidal anti-inflammatory drug (NSAID)? Use a heating pad or an ice pack? Do these things help or not? Write your answers down.

There's more you can do to fill out your pain profile, and every bit of information you enter into it will help your doctor help you. Other items to consider include whether the pain comes on suddenly or whether it's always present. Think back to the first time you felt the pain. What were you doing? Generally, it's easier to remember hurtful scenarios rather than good ones, which is helpful when it comes to medical diagnosis.

What are your other symptoms? Are you running a fever, or do you have diarrhea? Have you had an unexplained weight loss or feelings of nausea? Spend some time analyzing your total body health. By the end of the week, you'll have a good overview of what your pain profile is. You'll also have good information to take to that follow-up appointment with your pain specialist.

This may seem like a lot of work, but it's important. While the pain scale gives a baseline and information on how your pain changes during the day and from day to day, this scale is only one aspect of the whole picture. To get a complete picture of your pain experience, you also need to keep an activity log.

Keeping an Activity Log

How well can you function? That's the crucial question, so the next step is to jot down for the doctor the activities that you're able to do or not do. The more information you give your physician, the better she'll be able to help you. Your physician needs to understand how your pain is affecting your life. An activity log can give your doctors even more helpful information than telling them how much pain you are in.

The activity log keeps track of how much you are able to do on any given day. If an activity causes you pain or if you have to change what you're doing because of pain, that's essential information. For example, if your work requires you to lift, bend, or stoop, and these activities cause you pain, that's important. Your life is more than work, however, and recreation is essential to health. If you love to garden, knit, or play softball, and now you can't because of pain, that's important, too.

Combining the information on your pain scale with the information from your activity log will provide a complete picture of the impact pain is having on your life.

The Follow-Up Appointment

At your follow-up appointment, you and the doctor will review the results of your tests. You'll discuss your pain profile and your activity log and, with all this information at hand, devise a course of treatment. This treatment will focus on either curing the pain or finding ways to manage it.

The first scenario is always the preferred one, and many times, especially in cases of acute pain, it's definitely achievable. For chronic pain, however, a cure may not be a reasonable option. In this case, managing the pain so that it doesn't manage you becomes the treatment goal.

POINTERS ON PAIN

Sometimes you have concerns and want to seek a second or third opinion. Keep your pain specialist in the loop if you're considering this. It's professional and courteous.

Your physician has a wide variety of options to consider, and if the first one or two or even three choices aren't effective, it's important not to give up. There's always a way to make pain easier to live with.

In addition to medications, there are injections as well as surgical options. Physical therapy may provide the key to relief, and even simple lifestyle changes can bring welcome respite from pain. The following chapters cover each of these treatment possibilities.

The goal is to develop a pain game plan with your doctor. It is important that you comply with medication doses, physical therapy, and any other treatments that the plan entails. Appropriate follow-up on your part is crucial. If things are not working or if they seem to be getting worse with the current plan, check back with the doctor and make the necessary changes.

POINTERS ON PAIN

Purchase a small spiral notebook in which you can outline your goals for each appointment with your doctor. Write down all your questions for your physician before each visit. Leave space for the answers.

The Importance of Asking Questions

Make sure you have time to ask questions. Answering every conceivable question you may have will not happen in one meeting with your doctor. Having one to three questions on hand that you want to ask during each visit is probably a good start. But come prepared. It's easy to get distracted when you're in a doctor's office, which is why it may be easier for you to have your questions and concerns written down beforehand.

Pain can be devastating. By the time you go to a pain specialist, you probably have been in pain for several months to maybe even years. Your pain complaints have most likely gotten better and worse depending on many factors. People around you have seen you suffer. You may feel like a burden at times because things you can do for yourself and for others can be limited by pain. And, simply put, you're tired of dealing with the pain.

Following are some examples of normal questions you might ask your doctor, as well as some concerns you might express, grouped into categories, just as you did for the initial visit.

1. When will my pain go away? Will it ever go away?

2. Will surgery be my only option?

3. Will I end up in a wheelchair?

4. Can pain kill you?

5. Does getting old mean I will have pain?

6. Will my life ever become normal again?

7. Physical therapy is not working for me. I'm quitting.

8. My family thinks my pain is in my head. Others think that I'm making it all up.

9. I wish my family and co-workers would acknowledge that I am in pain.

The first six questions have to do with pain, the seventh statement is an evaluation of part of the treatment program, and the last two comments involve the psychological and emotional components of pain. All these questions and concerns are normal, and you and your pain specialist will work through them together.

Understanding Your Medications

Know what the purpose of each of your medications is and what your medication options are for your problems. It's common to think that medications are given to help relieve the pain. This is not always the case. In some cases, pain medications, such as opioids, are given to help you get through some physical activity or a challenging physical therapy session. Some nerve pain pills are given every day, even if you're doing all right that day, because they're needed to build up a therapeutic dosage level in your system to control chronic nerve pain. Understand what you're taking and why you're taking it. If you're not certain, get clarification from your doctor.

The Role of Physical or Occupational Therapy

Physical therapy is the hallmark of any pain management treatment plan, but it doesn't mean you have to see the physical therapist for the rest of your life. Therapy simply is a means to help you learn to use your body in the best way possible.

Often, doing physical therapy can cause some pain, which is expected. However, the exercises are meant to keep you functioning. They're to make sure that an injury in one place doesn't cause other parts of your body or your biomechanical system to break down. It's easy to see how a poorly managed ankle sprain can cause you to adopt an inappropriate walking pattern, resulting in long-term knee or back pain.

 STABS AND JABS

Don't quit your physical therapy sessions just because they hurt. Doing your physical therapy can hurt, but the goal is to improve your functionality, and sometimes getting to your goal requires some pain along the way. Physical therapy can help keep your pain from getting worse.

Nerve Injections

Many nerve blocks and injections are available to help treat pain. Make sure you keep a diary of all the injections you've gotten and when you got them. Jotting down notes on what worked and what didn't is also crucial. The generic term for all these injections is "nerve injections," so writing down the specific one you got can be important to your treatment plan.

Diagnostic Testing

Make sure you have a copy of your reports if not the full hard copy of the scans. Understanding your pain is often more than simply understanding your diagnostic tests, such as x-rays or MRI scans. If you have questions about these test results, talk to your doctor about your concerns. New tests are usually not necessary if your symptoms haven't changed, but if your doctor is planning on pursuing some new treatments, such as injections, further diagnostic testing may be indicated.

Follow-Up Appointments

Keep your follow-up appointments. It's easy to skip an appointment after an injection if the injection helped; however, follow-ups are important for both you and your doctor. They help your doctor evaluate the success of your treatment and help you keep on track with your pain plan. The best thing you can do for your health is to follow instructions and give accurate feedback so that the treatment plan can be changed when necessary or kept the same if it's working.

Following your pain management program requires patience and effort, but the results can empower you to live with increased functionality and less pain.

The Least You Need to Know

- A pain specialist is a physician with training in managing chronic pain.
- Developing your pain profile is the first step in creating a treatment plan.
- The goal of managing chronic pain is to increase your functionality.
- A psychologist or psychiatrist can help you cope with the psychological and emotional aspects of living with chronic pain.
- A pain log and an activity log give the best picture of how pain is affecting your life.
- Follow-up appointments are opportunities to ask questions about medications, procedures, or any topic related to your pain plan.

Medical Tests and Procedures

In This Chapter

- What your blood reveals
- When x-rays are in order
- The wide range of modern diagnostic options
- Fitting the procedure to your specific problem

Often medical tests and procedures are used to rule out specific causes for your pain if it's not apparent that your pain is the result of an injury. The good news is that you're probably already familiar with many of these tests and procedures. These may be done in the doctor's office, or you may be referred to a special imaging center. Imaging centers are often located close to major hospitals.

Blood Tests

A blood sample can be a routine part of a physical examination. Depending upon what's being tested, you may be asked not to take any food or drink for some hours prior to the blood draw. It is also very important to ask your doctor if you can take your regular medications before these types of tests.

The blood is usually taken from a vein on the inside of your arm around the crease between your upper arm and forearm. However, other sites can be used if needed. The nurse or technician will tie an elastic tourniquet around your upper arm and then use an antiseptic wipe at the place where the blood will be drawn. You may feel a slight pinch or sting as the collection needle is inserted.

Depending upon the tests to be run, the nurse will fill one or more test tubes. Then the nurse removes the needle and applies a dressing or sterile patch at the site. You'll leave this on for a short time—just to be sure there is no excessive bleeding at the site.

Sometimes slight bleeding continues under the skin after the needle is withdrawn. This can cause some bruising, called a hematoma, which disappears within a few days. Some medications that you may be taking (such as aspirin) can make you more susceptible to bruising.

There is a normal range of values for each test that is done. These values give information on the levels of certain proteins, blood levels of medications, or enzyme function. They can indicate whether your blood count is normal or whether any of your major organs, such as the liver or kidneys, show an infection or disease. Numbers that are outside the normal range, either higher or lower, can help your doctor home in on a diagnosis for your pain.

The most common blood test is called a CBC (Complete Blood Count). This test provides a wide spectrum of information. For example, a higher-than-normal white blood cell count can indicate infection or inflammation—a potential source of pain.

Your blood work reveals a great deal of information about the many organ systems in your body and how they are functioning. For example:

- Blood tests can help pinpoint pain resulting from a malfunctioning thyroid gland. This gland controls your metabolism. If it's overactive (hyperthyroid) or underactive (hypothyroid), you may experience a wide range of symptoms—from weight gain or weight loss to muscle aches and neuropathy (nerve pain).

- Another example is testing your blood sugar levels if you have diabetes. This test is called the HgbA1C. When your blood sugars are outside the normal range, you are at risk for many pain problems, including *neuropathies*.

- A C-reactive protein test looks for a specific protein (the C-reactive protein) in the liver, associated with inflammation.

Inflammation is a characteristic symptom of certain auto-immune diseases, such as lupus and rheumatoid arthritis. Inflammation is one of the ways your body responds when tissues are injured. Swelling, redness, pain, and heat are characteristic indications of inflammation.

 DEFINITION

Neuropathies are nerve disorders common in people with diabetes. Anywhere from 30 to 70 percent of diabetics will have nerve damage that can range from irritating to extremely painful.

Another test to see whether inflammation is present is called the erythrocyte sedimentation rate test or ESR. It's usually shortened to "sed rate." This test measures the length of time it takes for blood cells to settle to the bottom of a test tube. If the rate is higher than the normal rate, it may indicate inflammation, infection, or the presence of a chronic disease.

Other blood tests look to see whether you have certain genetic markers or antibodies. For example, the presence of an antibody called rheumatoid factor may indicate that rheumatoid arthritis is responsible for your pain.

The most important thing to remember about blood tests is that, often, taken by themselves, they may not mean anything. It is important to speak to your doctor about their relevance to you.

Imaging Tests

Imaging is just what the name implies—taking pictures, although these pictures concern structures such as bones, ligaments, tendons, and muscles inside your body. The equipment is sophisticated and uses state-of-the-art computer technology. Procedures are painless, and results are available instantly.

Some imaging procedures require you to either swallow or receive a contrast material by means of an intravenous (IV) drip. Depending upon the procedure, this contrast material may be a dye, barium sulfate (generally used for imaging of the digestive tract), or iodine-based. The contrast material enhances the images being taken. Before receiving the contrast material, inform the radiologist if you have had a reaction to contrast material in the past or if you are allergic to any of the following:

- Shellfish
- Barium
- Iodine
- Dyes
- Gadolinium

Also tell the radiologist if you have any of the following medical conditions:

- Asthma
- Diabetes

- Coronary artery disease

- Sickle cell anemia

- Kidney disease

- Multiple myeloma

- Pheochromocytoma (adrenal gland tumor)

These conditions can put you at risk for a reaction that can range from mild to severe. Severe reactions can include difficulty breathing and anaphylactic shock.

You should inform your physician of all medications you are taking. This includes over-the-counter drugs, vitamins, and supplements. For some imaging tests, you may need to discontinue medication use one to two days prior to imaging.

You'll be given detailed instructions for how to prepare for whatever imaging tests you'll be undergoing. Some will require you to fast for a certain number of hours before the test, while others will require you to increase your fluid intake prior to the test.

X-Rays

X-rays are a useful tool for discovering whether arthritis, bone fractures, or disc problems are causing your pain. They can also show whether you have an abnormal curvature of the spine.

An x-ray produces a two-dimensional picture. Radiography is the medical term for this diagnostic procedure, and it's the oldest imaging technique still in use today. In an x-ray, a bone fracture or other injury to bones, discs, or teeth can be seen. X-rays are not the best in detecting damage to soft tissues, however. X-rays can be frequently done on site at a doctor's office.

STABS AND JABS

X-rays can harm a fetus. It is essential to inform the radiology technician if you are pregnant or suspect you may be pregnant, so protective measures can be taken.

The principle behind x-rays is simple. A machine focuses a beam of electromagnetic rays at the site being photographed. This radiation is absorbed by your body to varying degrees, depending on the tissue being targeted. The picture is finished as a negative. Bone shows as white and other tissues as varying shades of gray or black.

Modern technology has reduced the amount of radiation dispatched with each picture taken, and this is good because overexposure to x-rays can damage cells. The effects of exposure to x-rays are cumulative. This is why you're given a lead apron when the pictures are taken. You want to protect as much of your body as possible.

CT Scan

A CT scan, also referred to as a CAT scan or computed tomography, uses x-rays to see whether damage to discs or other structures such as bones are responsible for your pain. These images are taken by the scanner and then sent to a computer, where they are translated into three-dimensional images. This technology is a definite improvement over the two-dimensional pictures generated by a traditional x-ray machine.

The machine is large and shaped rather like a donut. The camera is able to change angles, so the result is a series of pictures that can be pieced together to create the final result. This final result is called a tomogram.

Unlike a traditional x-ray, a CT scan can capture images of body organs. This can be helpful if an injury to an organ, infection, or a tumor is suspected of causing your pain. The procedure is totally painless. Occasionally it may be necessary to inject contrast material to get better definition on the pictures. This material is iodine-based.

You'll lie on your back on a special table that slides in and out of the scanner. You won't need to remove your clothing, and if you're cold, the technician can provide you with a light blanket.

The technician sits at a desk alongside the scanner and oversees the process. The table you're lying on then slides inside the scanner. There's a small mirror overhead so you can catch a glimpse of the room outside. During the picture-taking session, which can take up to an hour and a half, there will be times when the technician will ask you to hold perfectly still and hold your breath so that the picture isn't distorted by body movement.

You'll hear a series of clicks and snaps and whirring and other clanking sounds as the camera takes its series of pictures.

If you are claustrophobic, you can be given a mild sedative to reduce your anxiety. If at any time during the procedure you feel discomfort or anxiety, the technician is right there to assist you.

After the pictures have been taken, the table slides out of the scanner, and you're done. If you've been sedated, you will need to have someone drive you home.

Magnetic Resonance Imaging

A magnetic resonance imaging (MRI) scan may be used to gather more information after an x-ray has shown the source of a problem. It can also be helpful if other diagnostic scanning procedures, such as CT scans or sonograms, haven't been able to pinpoint the reason for your pain, and it's often used to see whether there's damage to nerves, muscle, or other connective tissue, internal organs, or bones. An MRI can also help find tumors or detect the presence of certain diseases.

An MRI uses different technology from traditional x-rays, and this means it doesn't use ionizing radiation. Instead, it uses a magnetic field and radio waves to obtain pictures, which are then sent to a computer. These pictures can be either two-dimensional slices, similar to the ones generated by a CT scan, or the computer can create three-dimensional pictures.

An MRI works by first creating a magnetic field around your body, and this in turn sets the water molecules in your body to moving about. While these water molecules are getting themselves back in position, radio waves are transmitted from the scanner and pass through your body, capturing the motion and sending it to a computer, which then turns out pictures of the area being examined.

STABS AND JABS

Don't get burned! Before undergoing an MRI, tell the technician if you have any tattoos. If the ink in the tattoo contains iron oxide, you can get a nasty burn at the site. The technician may place an ice pack over the tattoo to keep it cooled down during the scan and prevent burns to your skin.

Generally there is no preparation involved on your part. If you need to fast, you'll be informed of this at the time you schedule a scan.

Sometimes a contrast material will be needed to get clearer pictures. It can be injected into your bloodstream or given in a liquid that you swallow before the scan. During the scan, you'll be able to wear your street clothes, unless your clothing has a metal zipper or snaps. In that case, you'll need to wear that attractive paper garment provided by the facility.

You might be surprised at the items you'll be asked not to bring into the scanning room. Because the magnetic field is so strong, anything with metal can interfere with or be damaged during the scan. It's similar to passing through airport security. These items include:

- Eyeglasses
- Jewelry (including watches and any body piercings)
- Belts with buckles
- Keys
- Nail clippers and pocket knives
- Credit cards (because of the magnetic strip on the back)
- Bobby pins
- Partial bridges or other dental work that you can remove from your mouth
- Hearing aids

Not all metal is outside your body. Some of this metal doesn't pose any particular risk, although the technician may need to make adjustments for it. However, if you have a cochlear transplant, a pacemaker, a defibrillator, or have metal clips as a result of an aneurysm, you should not undergo an MRI. And if you have a pain pump or spinal cord stimulator in place, let your radiologist know.

STABS AND JABS

If you have any metal parts attached to your body, such as medical implants, screws, plates, or clamps, be sure to notify the technician before undergoing an MRI or a CT scan. Basically, if you weren't born with it, disclose it.

The machine itself is a large tubelike structure, and you'll lie on the table that's designed to slide in and out of the tube. A circular magnet around the machine creates the magnetic field.

As with the CT scan, you're going to be in an enclosed space, so if you aren't comfortable with this, you can be given a sedative to calm your nerves. Some MRIs are "open," which means the sides are not enclosed, and this can be helpful if you're claustrophobic.

Should you get an enclosed or "open" MRI? The "open" MRI pictures are often not as good as the enclosed MRI films. A discussion with your physician, taking into account your comfort level, what information she is looking for, and what the image will provide, is important to help you make this decision.

You'll need to lie as still as possible while the pictures are being taken. Fortunately this means just holding still for a few seconds to a few minutes at a time. Sometimes you may be asked to hold your breath for several seconds. This is to ensure good-quality shots. Also, as with the CT scan, you'll hear all sorts of interesting sounds—bumps and thumps and hums. If this bothers you, you can use foam earplugs.

You shouldn't feel discomfort, although sometimes the area that's being scanned can feel warm. If this happens, tell the technician. If you've had contrast material injected, you may feel flushed for a few minutes, but this passes quickly.

The scan generally takes from 45 minutes to an hour. Once the scan has been completed, the exam table slides out of the scanner. No specific aftercare is needed, and you'll be able to go about your normal activities. If you've taken a sedative, however, you'll need to have someone drive you home.

Electrodiagnostic Tests

Electrodiagnostic studies are made up of two parts: the electromyography test, abbreviated as EMG study (the needle study); and the nerve conduction study. This test helps provide information on whether there is a specific nerve injury present. Often, this study can help diagnose a pinched nerve, a general nerve problem, or other diseases that can cause neurological complaints.

This study uses a small needle that looks similar to an acupuncture needle. Although this study cannot damage your nerves, it can be mildly uncomfortable.

SPEAKING OF PAIN

You may not have thought of your body as producing electricity, but electrical impulses sent via your nervous system are what allow you to move your arms and legs.

In addition to injury, many medical conditions and diseases can cause pain due to nerve injury. These conditions include cancer, diabetes, and even vitamin deficiencies. Often, sciatica and carpal tunnel syndrome can be diagnosed through electrodiagnostic studies.

If you're experiencing nerve pain, you may be referred to a *physiatrist* or *neurologist*. Most often the physiatrist or neurologist will be able to conduct EMG or electrodiagnostic studies in the office to measure the electrical activity of the nerves.

DEFINITION

A **neurologist** is a physician who treats disorders of the nervous system. A **physiatrist** is a physical medicine and rehabilitation physician, otherwise known as a "PM&R" physician, who also treats disorders of the neuromuscular system.

During an EMG study, several electrodes will be placed on your skin to measure electrical impulses in the nerves. It's not a painful test, but you may feel some discomfort as the nerves are stimulated. You may feel a prick as small needles are placed in certain muscles. These needles are smaller than those used in taking blood samples. The first set of electrodes stimulates various nerves by giving a mild snap to the skin. The snap feels like a rubber band snapping, stimulating various nerves.

There's no special preparation involved on your part for EMG studies. You will most likely sit on the exam table and watch as the physician or technician places the electrodes on the areas to be studied. You may be asked to flex a muscle during the needle testing. Otherwise, you're a passive observer.

The procedure usually lasts around an hour. After the tests are completed, you can go about your normal activities. It is important to take all your medications on the day of the test and not wear any lotion, as the grease from the lotion can hinder the testing process.

Bone Scans

Bone scans are *nuclear radiology* procedures, used to detect the presence of infection in the bone, to find fractures that don't show up on regular x-rays, and to determine whether you may have arthritis or bone tumors. They're also used to monitor specific medical conditions, such as cancer. Essentially, they look for changes in the bone.

DEFINITION

Nuclear radiology is a field of radiology that uses radioactive material to send signals that can be recorded by a camera scanner.

For this procedure, a small amount of radioactive material is injected into a vein. If this material gathers at the spot where bone has been damaged, this gathering spot is called a "hot spot." The opposite, "cold spots," occur where the tracer isn't absorbed.

Both hot and cold spots can provide good diagnostic information. Then the scanner takes a picture of the hot spot, and the results are transmitted to a computer for analysis. Pictures can be taken at different intervals during the scan—for example, as the tracer is being injected, shortly afterward, and then up to several hours afterward.

There is no specific preparation for a bone scan, although if you are pregnant or nursing, be sure to tell your doctor who is ordering the test. The amount of radiation emitted by the tracer is small, but there is some risk of harm to the developing fetus, and the radioactive tracer can contaminate your breast milk, if you are nursing.

As with all types of scans, it's best to leave jewelry and other accessory items at home. You may be permitted to wear your street clothes during the scan, or you may be asked to put on a paper gown.

The technician will start an IV drip through which the tracer will be given. It takes anywhere from one to three hours for the tracer to collect at the site under study, so you won't have to be lying still the entire time.

You'll be given several glasses of water to flush the extra tracer from your system, so you'll want to remain close to the restroom during this time.

The actual scan takes about one hour. You'll empty your bladder one last time and then lie down on the exam table. You'll need to keep quite still, so the pictures will be clear. Then the scanner will move about your body, taking pictures. You may need to change positions during the procedure. After the scan is completed, the technician removes the IV, and you're free to go.

You'll be advised to increase your fluid intake for the rest of the day to ensure the tracer is completely flushed from your system.

Sonography

Sonography is also known as ultrasound, and its main purpose as a diagnostic tool is to discover injuries to muscles, ligaments, or tendons. During this procedure, sound waves sent from a transducer bounce back as echoes, after coming in contact with body tissues. These echoes create clear images of the area under study and send them to a computer for processing.

This procedure is usually done at an imaging center or as an outpatient service at the hospital. It's totally painless, and no preparation is required on your part. The procedure takes about half an hour.

First, the technician will apply a gel to your skin over the area to be examined. Then she'll pass the transducer, which resembles a hand-held wand, over the skin, and you can watch as the images show up on a video screen.

You may experience some pressure from time to time, as the technician presses more firmly at the area being studied.

 SPEAKING OF PAIN

People who are extremely obese may not be good candidates for ultrasound, as the body fat keeps the sound waves from going as deeply as they need to in order to get a good image.

After the procedure is completed, the technician will clean the gel from your skin, and you will be ready to resume your normal activities.

Discography

Discography is used to obtain images of the disc and to see if the disc is the reason for the pain. Discography is done when other procedures, such as x-ray or MRI, have been inconclusive or when the current pain treatment plan hasn't produced satisfactory results. It is often used to determine the extent of injury to the discs in the spine and is considered an *invasive procedure*. Some doctors consider it beneficial, and others disagree on its relative benefits.

During a discography, dye is injected into the center of a disc. If there are tears in the disc, the dye will dissipate throughout the area, and these tears can be captured on film. This type of testing is called a discogram. It is usually done under a *fluoroscope*.

It can also be done as part of a CT scan. This procedure is generally done at a special imaging center or a hospital and may take from half an hour to an hour to complete.

> **DEFINITION**
>
> An **invasive procedure** is the term used to describe any medical procedure that cuts through or enters the skin. It also refers to the insertion of any medical devices into the body. An injection is a minimally invasive procedure.
>
> A **fluoroscope** is a medical imaging device that provides real-time images of the bony parts of the body. It uses an x-ray source and a display screen. The x-rays pass through the individual and are displayed on the screen.

You will be awake during the procedure. You may be given a mild sedative before the procedure and IV sedation as well. If the pain area is in your upper back, lower back, or neck, you will generally lie on your stomach.

Your back will be wiped with an antiseptic to help prevent infection. Then the discs will be injected with the dye, which may also contain an antibiotic to further reduce the possibility of infection.

Injections into a normal disc will give the sensation of pressure but shouldn't be painful, and the physician will inject a normal disc with the dye to establish a baseline of comfort/discomfort. However, when the dye is injected into a damaged disc, you will feel some pain, and you will be asked to describe it. The physician should prepare you prior to the procedure on what types of questions you'll be asked, along with when and how they'll be asked to avoid any confusion during the procedure.

> **STABS AND JABS**
>
> Discography is not recommended for people who are actively taking blood-thinning medications. You should not undergo this procedure if you have an infection anywhere in your body, as complications can occur as a result.

Because you have received an anesthetic, you will need to have someone drive you home after the discography has been completed. You may feel some discomfort afterward, but this can be treated with ice packs and analgesics.

CT Myelography

This imaging procedure is used to examine the spinal cord and the spinal canal, along with the nerve roots and the blood vessels associated with these structures. If your physician suspects that the cause of your back pain is a ruptured or herniated disc, also called a slipped disc, she may order a CT myelogram to see if this disc is pushing on the spinal canal or nerve roots.

This procedure can also be used to confirm a diagnosis of narrowing of the spinal canal, a condition called spinal stenosis. In addition, it is used to check for infection, injury, tumors, or inflammation in this area. If surgery is being considered, a CT myelogram may provide important information about what needs to be done.

For this procedure, a needle is inserted into the spinal canal, and contrast material is delivered into the injection site. Fluoroscopy or CT scans are taken to be sure the needle is in the correct position. These scans show up on the computer screen in real time. Each picture that results is called a myelogram. Like discography, CT myelography is an invasive procedure.

Evaluating the Diagnostics

Blood work and imaging tests provide your physician and your surgeon with a great deal of information that cannot be gathered from your medical history or your explanation of your symptoms.

Sometimes your symptoms are saying the pain is coming from one place, when the problem is actually located quite some distance from where you're feeling it, or the pain is actually the result of an underlying medical condition.

POINTERS ON PAIN

You are a person with pain. You are more than numbers on a lab report. You are not a diagnosis. Sometimes you may feel that the process of discovering the source of your pain has become more important than you are. If this happens, speak up and tell your doctor how you are feeling.

Diagnostic blood work and imaging tests literally get beneath the surface to see what's really going on with your body. Still, they aren't foolproof, and that's why they need interpretation. Sometimes the tests may say one thing, but that one thing may not be correct. No test is infallible. And sometimes the results are inconclusive. Even when this happens, however, there is value in the test. Diagnosis is often about ruling out some possibilities in order to consider others.

The Least You Need to Know

- Each test in your blood work has a range of normal values. Your test results show where you fall in that range.
- X-rays are used to diagnose problems with bones, but soft tissues require other imaging tests.
- Sound waves, electrical impulses, and magnetic resonance can help home in on the source of your pain.
- Computerized diagnostic procedures give real-time diagnostic results.

Oral and Topical Medications

In This Chapter

- Finding the right medication for the job
- Common side effects of medications
- Avoiding double-dosing
- Safety precautions

Many medications, both over-the-counter as well as prescription types, are helpful in treating pain. Some work to relieve swelling and inflammation; others focus on pain relief. Some you take by mouth and some topically (by putting them directly on the area causing pain), which is a great alternative for children and adults who have a difficult time taking pills. In this chapter, we'll look at the medications most often recommended for treating pain.

Acetaminophen

Acetaminophen is an *analgesic* that has been around for more than half a century. It's often the first line of defense in treating sudden-onset pain. A common inhabitant in most people's medicine chests, acetaminophen is also a fever reducer. Tylenol is a brand of acetaminophen.

DEFINITION

An **analgesic** is a drug used for pain relief that may or may not have anti-inflammatory properties. It works by blocking pain receptors in the central nervous system.

Acetaminophen is helpful in relieving headache pain, low back pain, toothache, and pain associated with osteoarthritis. In general, most things that hurt can be helped by acetaminophen. It's generally safer for children than aspirin. Unlike some medications, you don't develop a tolerance to acetaminophen, and this means you don't need to keep increasing the dosage to achieve the same desired effect.

Acetaminophen comes in a variety of forms: tablets, gel-caps, liquid, or as suppositories. Although acetaminophen has proven to be generally safe for pregnant and nursing mothers, exceeding the recommended dosage can increase the risk of liver damage. Follow the recommended dosage instructions given to you by your doctor. Remember to tell your doctor if you take other medications and if you drink alcohol.

Side effects of acetaminophen use are uncommon but may include severe liver damage at high doses.

If you are giving this medication to your child, discontinue use after five days if no improvement is seen and contact your child's physician. There are exceptions to this rule, but in general it's a good way to proceed.

NSAIDs

NSAIDs (pronounced "N-sayds" or "N-seds") are a broad group of nonsteroidal anti-inflammatory drugs. As the name implies, NSAIDs do not contain *steroids* (such as prednisone, for example), which means they come without some of the side effects that long-term use of steroids can cause. NSAIDs have the basic pain-relieving properties of analgesics along with the ability to reduce inflammation.

DEFINITION

Steroids are a class of synthetic drugs that mimic the effects of cortisol, a naturally occurring hormone in the human body. Frequently referred to as corticosteroids or glucocorticoids, these drugs are not the same as the performance-enhancing steroids used by some athletes.

NSAIDs are used for treating arthritis pain, headache pain, muscle pain resulting from injury, and pain associated with menstrual cramps. They block certain enzymes in the body that create hormones. In the process, they also reduce inflammation.

POINTERS ON PAIN

Inflammation is the body's natural response to infection or injury. Suppressing that response for prolonged periods of time can be harmful, so it's important to follow dosage instructions carefully.

NSAIDs work by slowing down the production of prostaglandins, which are fatty-acid derivatives found in just about all of your organs and tissues. The two types of these prostaglandins are COX-1 and COX-2. NSAIDs are COX-1 and COX-2 inhibitors.

These prostaglandins have several important functions, among them sending pain messages to your central nervous system (CNS) and promoting inflammation and fever. That's good and bad.

It's good when you get the pain message and can do something about it, such as taking your hand away from the hot stove. It's not good when the pain message keeps repeating itself like a broken record, long after you've removed your hand from the heat.

It's good when fever and inflammation are part of the healing process, sending battalions of white blood cells to deal with injury and infection. It's not good when fever and inflammation continue after the problem has been resolved.

And that's where NSAIDs come into the picture, stopping those messages so you get pain relief. Many NSAIDs are available as over-the-counter medications or by prescription. Different NSAIDs have different degrees of strength and different potentials for side effects. Side effects range from the minor—nausea and upset stomach—to the serious—stomach ulcers, bleeding, stroke, and even cardiac problems.

NSAIDs also differ in how long the effects of each dose last and in the way they are eliminated from your body. In the following sections, we'll cover the NSAIDs most often used for pain relief.

Aspirin

It may come as a surprise, but the NSAID known as aspirin originally was a trademarked name. It lost its trademark early in the twentieth century, however, and has become a generic term for a drug that contains both pain-relieving and anti-inflammatory properties.

> **STABS AND JABS**
>
> Because of the risk of Reyes Syndrome, a potentially life-threatening condition linked to aspirin use in children and adolescents, these populations should not take aspirin.

Aspirin (acetylsalicylic acid) is available as an over-the-counter drug and in extended-release form as a prescription item. Aspirin purchased as over-the-counter medication is effective for relieving headaches, toothaches, muscle aches and pains, menstrual cramps, and osteoarthritis. As a prescription medication, aspirin is used to relieve the pain of rheumatoid arthritis and other rheumatologic conditions.

Aspirin comes in tablet form. The label will tell you whether the tablets are chewable or should be swallowed whole, with a full glass of water. Extended-release tablets should not be chewed.

Aspirin is used in some instances (such as prevention of heart attack) as a blood-thinner or anticoagulant, so if you're taking aspirin for these reasons, you should inform your physician before scheduling any type of surgery or minor procedures. Otherwise you risk excessive bleeding during and after surgery. Most surgeons will ask you to stop taking aspirin one to two weeks before scheduled surgery.

Follow the dosage instructions on the aspirin label carefully and do not exceed the recommended dosage. If you don't get pain relief within a few days, discontinue use of aspirin and consult your physician.

Common side effects of aspirin include nausea, upset stomach, and heartburn.

Ibuprofen

Ibuprofen is the generic name for an NSAID sold under several brand names, including Advil, Motrin, Nuprin, and Midol. It's a familiar medication, but it requires careful and intelligent use. This is a medication you don't want to use for an extended period of time, as it has been implicated in heart attack and stroke. It is also important not to exceed the recommended dosage while you are taking ibuprofen.

Some side effects of ibuprofen include:

- Nausea

- Stomach pain

- Heartburn
- Dizziness
- Rash
- Diarrhea
- Ringing in the ears

POINTERS ON PAIN

For a complete list of possible side effects of medications, read the label or insert that comes with that medication.

Naproxen

Naproxen is the generic term for an NSAID sold over the counter under brand names that include Aleve, Midol Extended Relief, and Naprosyn. It's also available by prescription.

Common side effects of naproxen include constipation or diarrhea, drowsiness, gas or heartburn, stomach upset, and stuffy nose.

Other commonly used NSAIDs include the following:

- Diclofenac (Voltaren)
- Diflunisal (Dolobid)
- Etodolac (Lodine)
- Indomethacin (Indocin)
- Ketoprofen (Orudis)
- Ketorolac (Toradol)
- Nabumetone (Relafen)
- Oxaprozin (Daypro)
- Piroxicam (Feldene)
- Salsalate (Amigesic)
- Sulindac (Clinoril)
- Tolmetin (Tolectin)

Each drug within the class of NSAIDs is different. Some are more powerful than others, but all have the potential for serious side effects (see "A Few Words of Warning" later in this chapter). If you have questions about drug interactions, or if you have concerns about side effects, ask your pharmacist or physician.

Common side effects of all NSAIDs include heartburn, nausea, bloating, stomach pain, vomiting, and dizziness.

COX-2 Selective Inhibitors

Thanks to television and magazine advertisements, we're much more aware of the names of specific new drugs than we used to be. Some of them have become household words. Celebrex is one such drug.

Celebrex is a COX-2 selective inhibitor. COX-2 selective inhibitors are a subset of the NSAIDs that suppress the production of the COX-2 prostaglandin. Celecoxib (Celebrex) is currently the only COX-2 selective inhibitor approved for use by the USDA. Other COX-2 selective inhibitors have been removed from the market because of their potential for serious side effects, which unfortunately include death.

Common side effects of Celebrex include the following:

- Constipation or diarrhea
- Gas or heartburn
- Nausea
- Sore throat
- Dizziness
- Stuffy nose

Muscle Relaxants

When you've injured your lower back, the resulting pain can also be accompanied by muscle spasms, some of which can be severe.

Muscle relaxants are often prescribed for this type of injury. However, these medications are sedatives, so you shouldn't take them if you're going to be driving, operating any kind of machinery, or need to be mentally alert. They're best taken just before bedtime.

Muscle relaxants act on the CNS to bring quick relief from spasms. They're prescribed for immediate and short-term use and generally aren't intended to address chronic pain, although they may sometimes be prescribed for long-term use in treating muscle spasms.

Medications with muscle relaxant properties include:

- Valium (diazepam)

- Zanaflex (tizanadine)

- Baclofen

- Flexeril (cyclobenzaprine)

Some of these medications can be tolerance-forming, so they're best used in small, effective dosages over the shortest period of time.

Common side effects of muscle relaxants include blurry or double vision, drowsiness, lightheadedness, or dizziness.

Opioids

Opioids are narcotics and are generally prescribed for acute pain. Sometimes they are also prescribed for treating chronic pain. They are analgesics, which means they provide pain relief, but they do not address inflammation. They work by blocking pain signals sent to the CNS.

Opioids are scheduled medications. This means that a special prescription is required for them. Oftentimes, these medications cannot be called in to the pharmacy but instead must be faxed by your doctor's office or taken to the pharmacy as a written prescription. Since they have the potential for building tolerance and causing serious side effects, it is essential to follow your physician's dosage instructions carefully and accurately.

POINTERS ON PAIN

Tylenol with codeine (acetaminophen with codeine) is available in Canada without a prescription. It is illegal to purchase it in Canada and bring it into the United States without a doctor's prescription.

Opioids may be prescribed as tablets, liquids, rectal formulations, or administered through injection or intravenous (IV) drip. Commonly used opioids to treat pain include the following:

- Acetaminophen with codeine (Tylenol with codeine)
- Hydrocodone with acetaminophen (Vicodin, Lorcet, Lortab)
- Oxycodone with acetaminophen (Percocet)
- Propoxyphene with acetaminophen (Darvocet)
- Morphine sulfate
- Oxycodone (OxyContin, Roxicodone)
- Propoxyphene (Darvon)
- Oxycodone with aspirin (Percodan)

You've probably noticed the frequent mention of acetaminophen in the preceding list. It's an ingredient in many over-the-counter and prescription combination drugs.

If you're already taking acetaminophen, be aware that doubling up on your intake of this drug can have serious consequences, including liver failure. Check with your pharmacist or your physician to be sure you are not overdosing yourself.

Common side effects of opioids include nausea, constipation, dizziness, urinary retention, sedation, and depressed mood.

Antineuropathic Pain Medications

Neuropathic pain occurs when the CNS and/or peripheral nervous system (PNS) doesn't work properly. This pain can be a result of injury or a medical condition (such as diabetes or cancer). Many times, the cause of nerve pain is not known. In some cases, this neuropathic pain becomes chronic. You may have heard this condition referred to as neuritis or neuralgia. Regardless of the name, the pain can be burning, shooting, stabbing, or hot.

 SPEAKING OF PAIN

According to the National Pain Foundation, about four million people in the United States suffer from neuropathic pain.

Neuropathic pain can be difficult to treat. Three kinds of medications are most generally used to treat neuropathic pain: local anesthetics, antidepressants, and anticonvulsants.

Local Anesthetics

Local anesthetics can be given intravenously, applied as a patch, or worked into the skin as a gel. They provide pain relief by deadening the nerve endings. They work similarly to the medications your dentist uses to numb your gums prior to dental work. Lidocaine, mexiletine, and bupivacaine are commonly used local anesthetics.

Common side effects include allergic reactions, such as itching, hives, or swelling at the site of the injection.

Antidepressants

Often, medications have the ability to treat a variety of symptoms. This is the case with antidepressants, which have the ability to relieve pain at fairly low dosages. For treating neuropathic pain, an older type of antidepressants, called tricyclics (TCAS), are most often prescribed. Nortriptiline and Amitriptyline are commonly prescribed tricyclic antidepressants.

Common side effects of antidepressants include nausea, dry mouth, urinary retention, fatigue, sleepiness or insomnia, blurred vision, agitation, and weight gain.

Anticonvulsants

As with antidepressants, anticonvulsant medications have proven effective in treating neuropathic pain. They reduce the intensity of pain signals originating in the brain and calm the nerves.

If you think about it, the brain and spinal cord are the biggest "nerves" in your body. Therefore, if anticonvulsants help the brain to decrease abnormal firing, such as happens when a person has a seizure, then (in lower doses) they can help other nerves decrease their firing and therefore decrease pain.

Gabapentin (Neurontin), carbamazepine (Tegretol), Lamictal, Keppra, and Topomax are commonly prescribed anticonvulsant medications used in treating neuropathic pain.

Your physician may prescribe one or more drugs from these categories, since combining these medications can often provide the most relief.

Common side effects of anticonvulsants include dizziness, constipation, and drowsiness.

Creams and Gels

There's definitely something soothing about applying a topical lotion, cream, or gel to your skin. Just the action of squeezing out the substance and then rubbing it in ever so gently seems to convey comfort. How exactly do these items work?

The answer is that they work in two different ways—they either promote sensations of coolness or sensations of heat. Both sensations essentially change what's going on with your sensory nerves, giving them something else to focus on, so the result is relief.

It might seem counterintuitive, but applying a cream that contains the substance that makes hot peppers hot (capsaicin) to your skin can give you pain relief. Capsaicin works by acting on a substance (called Substance P) found in the nerve cells in your skin, disrupting its ability to transmit pain signals to your CNS. These creams include the following:

- Zostrix
- Arthricare
- Capzasin

Other topicals that use wintergreen, eucalyptus oil or menthol work as counter-irritants. That means they create sensations of heat or coolness on your skin. These creams include the following:

- Icy Hot
- JointFlex
- Flexall 454

Experts disagree on the effectiveness of topical preparations, but some people are convinced they work. In any case, the effect of topical applications is temporary.

Common side effects of topical preparations include rash.

A Few Words of Warning

Medications can be extremely effective in relieving different types of pain, but you need to be aware of certain basic cautions. Some of these cautions center on proper use, and others on how to obtain these drugs.

The first rule is to not stop any medication abruptly unless you've checked first with your doctor and have been told to do so. Often, these medications need to be weaned down over time to reduce side effects and keep you safe.

Overusing Pain Medications

If a little is good, is more better? The answer is not necessarily. Each medication has a therapeutic dosage, which means there's an optimal level at which that drug does its best work. Go under that level, and you don't get much relief. Go beyond that level, and you risk some serious harm from overdosing and/or side effects. In some cases, overdosing can be lethal.

General guidelines have been developed that show the amount of medication that may be effective for treating pain. That said, all individuals have their "therapeutic" dosages that work for them. This amount varies greatly, depending on a person's own body and reactions to the medication. Each of us is different, and we all react differently to medication.

Familiarity breeds contempt, or at least a casual attitude. When this attitude extends to your medications, it can be dangerous. This warning applies to over-the-counter medications, as well as to prescription items.

SPEAKING OF PAIN

Unintentional overdoses of products containing acetaminophen, such as Tylenol, account for up to 25 percent of acute liver failure cases in the United States each year.

Your liver works hard at metabolizing the various substances you ingest on a daily basis. From food to alcohol to medications, it has a wide range of responsibilities. In the case of medications, taking too much of a drug, such as one that contains acetaminophen, can tax your liver to the max and permanently damage liver cells. The result can be acute liver failure, definitely something you want to avoid.

Since more than 100 over-the-counter products contain acetaminophen, it can be very easy to exceed the correct dosage. You can find acetaminophen in the following over-the-counter preparations:

1. Cold and flu medications

2. Headache medications

3. Sinus medications

4. Sleep aids

5. Menstrual cramp remedies

Read the label before you take any medication. Know what you're taking and follow the dosage directions accurately, even when taking common over-the-counter medications, and you'll reduce your chances of developing a possibly fatal complication.

Alcohol and Pain Medications

A glass of wine, a shot of the hard stuff, or a bottle of beer are age-old remedies for what ails you. And it's definitely true that alcohol can dull a nagging ache or pain, at least for a short period of time. However, alcohol is a depressant, and you can build up your tolerance to it so that it takes more and more to give you relief. And it's not a cure. It can become a serious problem if you decide to mix drinks and pain medications.

Now that you've gotten the good habit of reading the labels on your medications (both over-the-counter and prescription), you'll notice that some tell you not to drink alcohol while taking that drug. Why?

It's back to your liver again, and this time with the added problem of developing stomach ulcers and bleeding. In the case of combining alcohol with certain narcotics (such as codeine or Darvon, among others), you risk possibly fatal consequences because your CNS can shut down.

The bottom line? If you're taking pain medications, don't drink alcohol, even in moderation, unless your physician says it's alright to do so.

Buying Medications over the Internet

It's convenient to purchase medications over the Internet, but be sure the site you are using is legitimate and that you are filling a valid prescription. There are scams galore on the Internet, and you want to be sure you're not the next victim.

Legitimate sites will have a licensed pharmacist on hand to be sure you're getting the correct prescription and will also be available to answer questions concerning your medications. These legitimate sites also offer a telephone option. So first try them out by calling them.

To be sure the site you're using is legitimate, check it out with the National Association of Boards of Pharmacy before you give out your credit card number. You can find them at www.nabp.net.

 STABS AND JABS

The U.S. Department of Justice Drug Enforcement Agency (DEA) is cracking down on individuals who buy controlled substances (narcotics) over the Internet without a valid prescription. This is illegal and extremely dangerous. Know the law!

Buying Medications Outside the United States

Medications are expensive, and insurance plans don't often cover all or even part of their cost. As a result, you may be tempted to purchase your medications from another country, such as Mexico or Canada.

Many of these medications are safe. Many may not be, and the appearance of the packaging is not a clue. Sometimes the labeling looks legitimate but isn't. Some of these medications do not contain the drug you think you're buying. Some do not contain it in the amount specified on the label. And some may contain harmful fillers and other agents that can put your health in jeopardy. It's a risky business.

The USDA is your backup regarding quality, cleanliness, and content of the medication you're using. However, their jurisdiction stops at the border. They have no power of regulation or enforcement outside the United States. Bottom line: be aware of the risks while you're considering the potential benefits of purchasing your drugs from another country.

Sharing Medications

Sharing prescription medications is never a good idea. You may be unaware of the other person's medical history, and your good deed may result in that person experiencing serious or potentially fatal side effects. Allergies, side effects, or the exact opposite—no effect at all—all are reasons not to share.

STABS AND JABS

Protect your medicines! Store them properly. A cool, dry location is best. Bathrooms can get hot and steamy—the worst possible conditions for storing medications. Use a closet or shelf away from the bathroom and always keep them away from children.

Expiration Dates

You'll find an expiration date somewhere on the label of your over-the-counter or prescription medications. What is an expiration date, exactly?

If you are a drug manufacturer and want FDA approval for your new drug, you'll conduct tests on it to see how it holds up over time. You don't want it to break down, change its composition, or do anything else that will compromise its structural integrity and potency. So you test it for a certain length of time. Then, when it's time to get the drug on the market, you indicate that the drug held up for one or two years—whatever the length of the test period.

The expiration date simply tells you that the manufacturer's testing procedures for that drug confirmed its strength and stability for a specific period of time. It doesn't mean that Drug X will crash and burn the day after the expiration date. It simply means it hasn't been tested beyond that point.

What this means is that, first of all, you should take your medications as prescribed—for the full course of treatment as indicated by your physician. That would eliminate a considerable amount of outdated drugs hanging around your home.

With the exception of medications that need to be refrigerated, such as liquid antibiotics, insulin, and so forth, the medication is most likely still fine. You just can't be 100 percent sure about its effectiveness.

So if you've bruised your knee, have a toothache, or your bursitis is acting up again, you're probably just fine if the expiration date isn't too far in the distant past. For serious conditions, check with your pharmacist and be safe. That may mean getting a refill to keep you current.

The Least You Need to Know

- Acetaminophen works well for most minor aches and pains.
- NSAIDs combine the properties of pain relievers and anti-inflammatory medications.
- Topical medications work by creating a counter-sensation of heat or cold and redirecting pain sensors in your skin and your brain.
- Your body can build up a tolerance to opioids in a few weeks of usage, so these medications are best used for short periods of time in the smallest effective dosages.
- Difficult-to-treat neuropathic pain, common with diabetes, may respond well to local anesthetics, antidepressants, or anticonvulsant medications.
- Many medications do not mix well with alcohol. Check with your doctor before you imbibe to avoid mixing a potentially fatal cocktail.

Medications Through Injections

In This Chapter

- Quick relief for pain
- Calming irritated nerves
- Relaxing knotted muscles
- Self-regulating your medications

Injections work in two ways. They can deliver medications, such as anesthetics and sometimes cortisone, directly to the painful area. Relief can be immediate or delayed, although often it's not permanent. Some injections work to block the "pain in the brain" pathway that we talked about in Chapter 1. This is especially true for pain problems lasting one month or longer, which we call chronic pain. In this chapter, we'll examine the different types of injections administered for pain relief.

Common Joint Injections

Local injections of corticosteroids can be useful in treating trigger finger, carpal tunnel at the wrist, and tennis elbow or tendinitis (see Chapter 13). Cortisone is a corticosteroid and frequently used for these injections. Other sites where these injections may be beneficial include the following:

- Shoulder—for arthritis, rotator cuff tendinitis, bursitis

- Knee—for arthritis, bursitis

- Hip—for arthritis, bursitis

- Heel or arch of the foot—for plantar fasciitis

You may have heard that doctors won't inject cortisone into a joint more than three times over the entire course of your life. Three has become sort of the magic number for this type of injection. One injection into the joint can be beneficial—reducing inflammation and allowing healing to take place.

Repeated injections, however, have been shown to have the exact opposite result. Studies show that where corticosteroids are concerned, more is not better. Repeated injections into the joint can actually damage the tendons, weaken ligaments and cartilage, and slow the healing process.

This means that whether you've gotten relief with one injection or not, it's time to look at physical therapy and other treatment options to prevent a recurrence of your joint problem.

An injection delivers the medication directly to where it's needed, so it can get to work quickly. Since the medication isn't taken by mouth, side effects associated with the digestive system, such as stomach irritation, are circumvented.

STABS AND JABS

Cortisone can cause a temporary rise in blood sugar levels, so if you have diabetes you should consult with your physician before receiving an injection of a corticosteroid. The same advice holds true if you have an active infection. Cortisone can interfere with the body's immune response.

How It's Done

The skin surface above the joint is cleaned with an antiseptic solution. Then, in many cases, a needle is inserted into the space of the joint, and any extra fluid there is withdrawn by the needle and can be sent to the lab for analysis. After that, the medication is injected into the joint. The needle is withdrawn, and a small dressing is placed over the site of the injection.

Benefits and Risks

You may feel pressure or some stinging at the injection site. This is temporary. You should begin to feel relief within a few days. The procedure is generally considered safe with few side effects. These may include slight swelling or bruising at the injection site.

Nerve Blocks

Time out for a little rest and relaxation. That's basically what nerve blocks can do for your overworked nerve pathways. Sensations travel along these nerve pathways from various parts of your body to your brain so that you can decide to either enjoy the sensation if it's pleasurable or do something about it if it's painful. When the message is pain for a prolonged period of time, it's time to consider some options. Nerve blocks are one of those options.

Nerve block is a general term for several types of injections. Sometimes these injections are given to the neck, as well as to the upper or lower back. Since nerves are housed all over your body, some medical providers use the term "nerve block" to describe injections delivered in any area of the body—spine, shoulder, hips, and so on.

What nerve blocks have in common is that these injections use medications such as anti-inflammatory medications, local anesthetics, or a combination of both and are delivered near a specific nerve that may be causing you pain. Other medications can also be delivered in the nerve block but are less common. Often botox or clonidine is also put in nerve injections. The anesthetic or medication doesn't remain permanently at the point of injection. It is eliminated from your body over the course of several hours up to a few weeks. In that time, however, the cycle of pain may get a break, and so do you. That's the theory behind these injections.

Nerve blocks serve a variety of functions. They were originally used as diagnostic tools, to find the source of pain. The thinking went something like this: if no one was able to find the cause of the pain, perhaps making an educated guess was the way to go.

This meant deciding which nerve *might* be the culprit and then blocking that nerve from acting up. If the block brought pain relief, that was terrific, and the best possible outcome. If it didn't bring pain relief, at least it eliminated one possibility.

Types of Nerve Blocks

There are different categories of nerve blocks and different types of nerve blocks within those categories.

First of all, nerve blocks can be used to discover where the pain is coming from. When the source of the pain has been determined, subsequent nerve blocks can predict if anesthetizing that nerve will solve the problem or if surgery might be a better way to go. An additional purpose for nerve blocks is to head off a problem before it begins, and they are used to help decrease pain during surgery or minimize pain after.

POINTERS ON PAIN

If you are taking blood thinners or have a medical condition that affects your blood's ability to clot, talk with your physician before undergoing a nerve block.

Nerve blocks can be used on various areas of the body. The blocks that target specific areas on the head include the face, forehead, scalp, eyelids, upper jaw, nose, and palate.

Nerve blocks can also be used on the neck, shoulders, back, elbow, wrist, abdomen, pelvis, groin, legs, and feet.

How It's Done

In most cases, you'll report to the hospital or clinic as an outpatient. The procedure takes just a few minutes. If you're having the block done on your elbow or wrist, you may be asked to sit; otherwise you'll lie down on the surgical table.

There's a bit of a dress rehearsal before the actual procedure. The doctor will most likely do a test block using a local anesthetic. If the results are good, then the show goes on, using corticosteroids, alcohol, or phenol for the actual nerve block.

The doctor will insert the needle as close as possible to the troublesome area. Sometimes these nerve blocks are done under *fluoroscopy* or CT scanners or ultrasound machines to help the physician locate the correct anatomical area.

DEFINITION

Fluoroscopy is a procedure that uses x-rays to observe the body's bony structures in real time.

You may feel a sting or pinch as the needle is inserted. Ask the doctor before the start of the procedure whether she needs you to give her any information. Often the physician will give you instructions such as, "Tell me if the pain goes down your leg." This type of data helps to adjust needles if needed during the procedure.

After the right spot has been determined, the medication is dispersed and spreads near the nerve.

Then the needle is withdrawn, and you'll rest for a half hour or more before being discharged. You may or may not feel immediate relief, but remember that it generally isn't permanent relief.

Benefits and Risks

Nerve blocks can provide effective, if temporary, pain relief and break the cycle of pain. They can be especially helpful in dealing with cancer pain, particularly with advanced cancers, including pancreatic cancer.

There are risks associated with nerve blocks. Some are minor, and others are serious. Risks include the following:

- Soreness, bleeding, and itching at the injection site

- Rash

- Infection

- Increased pain

- Elevated blood sugar levels

- Nerve damage

Nerve blocks come with the potential for serious, and in rare cases, life-threatening complications. If the injection is delivered to the wrong nerve, it will not have the intended beneficial effect. If the injection misses its mark, the medication can be delivered into the bloodstream, instead of the targeted nerve. If the medication or needle goes into an artery, it can damage it.

Depending on the injection, complications can include loss of bowel and bladder function, paralysis, and weakness in the arms or feet. Other complications include the risk of a punctured lung, severely reduced blood pressure (a condition called hypotension), and in rare instances, death.

Trigger Point Injections and Tender Point Injections

Sometimes muscles forget how to relax. They knot up, and those knots are called tender points. They hurt. If these knots are close to the surface, you can feel them by running your fingers along your skin. They often feel rubbery under your fingers. Other times they are deeper, and you can't feel them, but they let you know they're there just the same.

Like tender points, trigger points are also very irritated spots on your body associated with tight muscle bands. The difference between tender points and trigger points is that trigger points can cause pain that is not just at the area of those tight muscle bands but can move from these areas into broader areas around those tender spots.

Trigger and tender points may result from injury to a muscle or muscle group or as a result of repetitive motions or incorrect posture that produce muscle strain and fatigue.

Injecting the trigger and tender points breaks up the muscle clumps. It may stop the trigger points from irritating the surrounding nerves and thus break the pain cycle. Sometimes a local anesthetic is injected into the muscle. Often, "dry needling," meaning no medications accompany the injection, helps more than an injection with an anesthetic.

SPEAKING OF PAIN

"Jump sign" is a way of finding out if there is a trigger point. If pinching a certain location makes someone forcefully pull away (jump), then most likely a trigger point was contacted and irritated. The reaction is much more severe than with someone who simply pulls away from a little pinch.

Trigger and tender points can occur in any muscle group, so this type of injection is often used for muscles in the back, neck, and shoulders. It's also used to treat the pain of fibromyalgia, low back pain, neck pain, and tension headache, to name a few conditions.

How It's Done

The injections can be done in the doctor's office or at the hospital or clinic. The area to be targeted is first cleansed with an antiseptic or alcohol swabs.

The needle then is inserted directly into the area of pain, and a local anesthetic is injected. Some physicians don't put any solution in the needle. The dry needling technique has shown effectiveness in relieving those darn knots. The muscle may twitch up to a few minutes after the needle is withdrawn, but relief can be instantaneous.

Your physician may recommend physical therapy to "re-educate" the muscles involved in the trigger point and prevent a recurrence. What's really important is to be compliant with a home exercise program as those muscles can be stubborn and can knot up again.

Benefits and Risks

Trigger point injections can provide immediate relief but may not be long-lasting. Complications can include swelling and bruising. A punctured lung is an uncommon complication, if the injection is delivered to a muscle near the rib cage.

Radiofrequency Ablation

In radiofrequency ablation, an electric current generated by a radio wave is targeted at a very small area of a nerve. This current destroys the cells that are causing pain or disrupting normal nerve pathway function.

This is a common procedure used to treat rapid, irregular heartbeat—a condition known as tachyarrhythmia. It's also used for low back and neck pain and has been helpful in relieving the pain of arthritis.

How It's Done

The procedure is usually done on an outpatient basis. You'll be given a sedative and a local anesthetic, since you need to be awake during the procedure to confirm when the correct spot has been reached.

Using fluoroscopy or CT scan for guidance, the surgeon inserts a *catheter* into the targeted area. When that's in place, a specialized needle is inserted through the catheter, and some preliminary electrical stimulation lets the surgeon know she's in the correct spot. Then the ablation is done. The needle tip delivers a local anesthetic and then an electric current to heat the nerves, thus disabling them. The positive effects can last a long time.

> **DEFINITION**
>
> A **catheter** is a hollow, flexible tube that can be inserted into a blood vessel or body cavity. It's used to deliver fluids or medications or allow removal of blood or other body fluids for testing. It can also be used to widen a narrowed passageway.

During the procedure you may feel some aching, tingling, or pain that is similar to the pain you've been experiencing. You will be awake for the procedure and asked to participate by answering simple questions that the physician may have for you while doing the procedure. Again, this helps her know that she is in the right place. The needle is then withdrawn, and a small dressing is taped to the skin over the incision.

Benefits and Risks

Radiofrequency is generally considered to be a safe procedure with minimal side effects.

Side effects can include soreness and bruising at the site. It also carries with it the same minor and major risk profiles as with any other nerve block discussed earlier.

Spinal Cord Stimulation

Spinal Cord Stimulation (SCS) is an implant procedure (also known as a dorsal column stimulator) that's used when some other pain relief procedures haven't done the trick for chronic or nerve-related pain. It's also performed when spinal surgery hasn't produced pain-relieving results.

The concept of a spinal cord stimulator is simple, even though the technology is complex. Think about how it feels when you burn your hand on a hot stove. Your first instinct is to pull your hand away from the stove. The second thing you do is rub the burnt hand with your other hand. Somehow this simple act of rubbing the injured hand decreases the sting of the burn. Essentially, the spinal cord stimulator acts the same way. It decreases pain by adding another sensation to the mix. It's a time-tested theory in pain management and is called the Gate Control Theory of Pain.

Technically speaking, the SCS produces a low-voltage electric current that the patient is able to turn on and off as needed. When the stimulator is turned on, it sends an electric impulse to the spinal cord, resulting in a tingling sensation.

The stimulator is battery-powered, and the batteries have a life span of two to five years, depending upon use. It's a package deal and comes with a remote-control (sort of like the one you use for your television) that you operate by hand to turn the stimulator on and off and regulate the strength of the impulses.

POINTERS ON PAIN

Spinal cord stimulation requires you to be very compliant with doctor evaluations and follow-ups. The device is implanted in your body, after all.

How It's Done

The procedure is a two-step process. First you'll receive a trial run to see whether SCS is the best way to treat your pain. You'll report to the hospital or clinic as an outpatient. You'll be given a local anesthetic, and then the physician will place a needle in the skin in some area of the neck, upper back, or lower back and insert a trial lead or wires through the hole of the needle.

The wire is then directed into the spinal canal around the area where the physician would like it to be placed.

Then you and your physician will decide if the area that hurts you is being stimulated. After that's been settled, you'll be given instructions in how to operate the stimulator. Each person's schedule is different, of course, but you can expect to use it several times a day or more.

When you completely know what to do, you'll be discharged. Many times, you will leave with the trial leads in place and be given specific instructions on when to come back to the doctor to have the leads pulled out. This will give you an opportunity to see if the stimulator works for you over the course of some days.

Benefits and Risks

Spinal cord stimulation provides pain relief when other measures haven't been effective. It doesn't eliminate the pain, however, but decreases it with a tingling sensation. This stimulation may not be comfortable for some people. If you decide you don't like the sensation produced, the implant can be removed or not even placed after the trial.

POINTERS ON PAIN

As long as you have a spinal cord stimulator in place, you can't get an MRI.

The stimulator has been effective in treating chronic pain that's related to a variety of medical conditions, including vascular disease, such as angina, and complex regional pain syndrome.

Complications can include the following:

- Scar tissue developing at the site of the stimulator
- Mechanical failure of the stimulator
- Infection
- Bladder problems
- Headache
- Spinal fluid leakage
- Decreased effectiveness of the stimulator as the body adjusts to it
- Pain spreading beyond the range of the stimulator

Spinal cord stimulation can be an effective tool for helping you tolerate chronic pain. You'll actually become your own programmer! Remember to turn off the stimulator when you pass through any theft detection devices, as they can cause your stimulator to spike. Also, carry your Implanted Device security card with you when you travel, as your stimulator will register at airport security.

Pain Pumps

Pain pumps, or implanted drug-delivery systems, send pain-relieving medications into your body near your spinal column. They are most often used to manage cancer pain and are helpful when other methods haven't been effective.

The pain pump itself is a hollow, round, metal device. Medication is stored inside the device, which is about the size of a hockey puck. A catheter leads from the pump to the area of the spinal column, where it can deliver the medication from the pump.

How It's Done

This procedure is done on an outpatient or inpatient basis. You'll be anesthetized. The surgeon makes an incision in your back and inserts a needle into that incision. She then sets the catheter in place via the needle. The medication will be delivered to this spot. Next, an extension catheter is positioned under your skin all the way from your back to your abdomen.

At this point, the surgeon makes another incision, inserts the pain pump, and attaches the catheter to it. This pocket where the pump will be placed can be put in the abdominal area or the buttocks. During the entire procedure, fluoroscopy or CT scans guide the surgeon's hands.

After everything is in place, the incisions are closed and covered with a dressing. You are shown how to use the pain pump, which must be refilled with medication as needed. The pump is programmed like a small computer to dispense medication on a specific schedule. This schedule can be modified as necessary.

After you've healed, your physician may refer you for physical therapy to help you learn how to exercise and go about your daily routine without injuring the pump or yourself.

Benefits and Risks

It is important to remember that this procedure, like the spinal cord stimulator, is surgery. The pain pump takes the place of oral medications, so that you get better pain relief with fewer side effects. It's got a good success rate in treating cancer pain.

Risks include the normal risks associated with surgery: infection, bleeding, and swelling at the surgical site. Since the surgical site is so close to the spinal column, there is some risk of leakage of cerebral spinal fluid, neurological injury, or bleeding in the spinal column. These potential risks can be serious and, in some cases, life-threatening.

The pain pump is a mechanical device, and machines can break. If the machine malfunctions or the catheter springs a leak, an overdose of medication can occur. The machine can also stop working and deliver no medication to you.

The Least You Need to Know

- Nerve blocks are injections that can deliver medication directly to a specific area, causing pain relief.
- Implants are surgical procedures that can provide ongoing relief for serious pain.

- Electrical current can be used to destroy specific nerve cells responsible for pain.
- A pain pump can be effective for managing cancer pain.
- All medical procedures come with an element of risk. Before you decide on a course of action, weigh the pros and cons carefully and discuss your decision with your surgeon or physician.

Physical and Occupational Therapy

In This Chapter

- Strengthening muscles for pain relief
- Working out at home
- Active and passive therapies
- Using assistive devices

Physical therapy can get you back in motion again, and occupational therapy can give you the tools to accomplish your goals. Often, when you feel pain, your first response is to limit your activity, rather than risk causing the pain to increase in intensity. That's just the opposite of what you should be doing in most cases. To help you learn the right way to move, your doctor may refer you to therapy. Often, physical therapy is combined with nerve blocks to get the best outcome and pain control.

About Physical Therapy

Physical therapy is designed to restore function and improve mobility when illness or injury has caused a disability. Physical therapy can help with pain relief, but sometimes that's not the primary reason for working with a physical therapist.

Sometimes the goal of physical therapy is to maintain good functioning in the rest of your body—the parts that can help you cope with where it hurts. For example, if you have knee arthritis, your physician may refer you to physical therapy so you learn how to strengthen your quadriceps muscle and stretch your hamstring muscles, which can tighten up with knee pain.

Improving muscle function may not always give you pain relief in the short term, but it can definitely help keep you functional for the long haul, whether you are pain-free or not.

What Physical Therapists Do

Physical therapists deal with a wide range of pain issues. From helping you learn how to live with chronic pain, to working with you to learn how to use replacement joints, to teaching you ways to prevent low back pain, your physical therapist is a key member of your health-care team.

A physical therapist can do much more than show you how to move without making matters worse. She can also show you the right way to move and to exercise to get the upper hand on pain. In many cases, physical therapy can postpone or even negate the need for surgery.

If you're recovering from a fracture or muscle injury or have a medical condition, such as multiple sclerosis, that causes pain, your physical therapist will work with you to strengthen muscles and increase your range of motion and flexibility—all important factors in relieving pain.

> **SPEAKING OF PAIN**
>
> Physical therapists practice in a variety of settings, including hospitals, clinics, and private facilities. They are licensed by the state in which they practice. One of their professional organizations is the American Physical Therapy Association.

Insurance Coverage

Your insurance company may cover part or even all of the cost of physical therapy, but it may have specific requirements you'll need to follow. Check with your carrier before you make your first appointment to see what these requirements are.

Ask your insurance carrier if a physician referral is required before they will make payment or if you'll be covered if you schedule your physical therapy without a referral. Also find out whether you can choose your own physical therapist or if you must select one from a list of preferred providers.

If you decide to select your own physical therapist instead of using a preferred provider, be sure to find out whether the claims your therapist submits on your behalf will be honored by your carrier.

Your First Appointment

At your first appointment you'll meet your therapist and spend some time discussing your concerns and what you hope to achieve with physical therapy. You'll fill out a questionnaire to give your therapist some basic information, and then the therapist will conduct some tests and take some measurements to determine the current levels of your range of movement, flexibility, and strength. After this data has been gathered, you and the therapist will develop a plan for your therapy.

POINTERS ON PAIN

Your physical therapy plan will include goals, a timetable for reaching these goals, and "homework"—exercises you will do at home to supplement your therapy.

The goal is not to have you in therapy forever. You and your therapist will decide on a reasonable course of therapy that may last one week or one month, for starters. After that you'll reappraise your goals and see if further therapy is needed or if you can continue on your own at home. Each therapy session will generally last from 30 minutes to an hour and will usually be a mix of active and passive therapies.

What to Wear

Dress down. Wear clothes that allow you to move freely. That means loose and comfortable. T-shirts and shorts or sweats are the best choices. Athletic shoes and socks complete your physical therapy wardrobe. Leave the jewelry at home. Some physical therapy sites have lockers available for storing personal items while you're in session, but others don't. The less extra stuff you have with you, the more you'll be able to focus on your therapy as opposed to wondering where you left your purse or your computer bag.

Practice Makes Perfect

Undergoing physical therapy is quite a bit like learning to play a musical instrument or a sport. You get out of it what you put into it. If you don't practice and just go to your lessons, you're not going to go very far. If you just go to your physical therapy sessions but don't follow through at home, you're not making the best use of this resource.

Keep a positive attitude. You are not a passive observer in your therapy, but an active participant. The closer you follow your regimen and the more faithfully you keep to your schedule, the better results you'll achieve.

Sometimes what seemed clear when you were working through an exercise at your therapy session isn't all that clear when you're practicing on your own. It's helpful to keep a small notebook handy while you're doing your homework so you can jot down concerns and questions as they arise. Take this to your next session and get those issues addressed.

Passive Therapy

We said previously that you're an active participant in your physical therapy, and that's true. However, at certain times in your session, the therapist will be doing the work. Some of this you won't be able to do on your own, so take advantage of it for as long as your sessions continue.

Passive therapies are used generally before and after the active portion of your session. They help prepare your muscles for exercising so you don't injure them. These treatments also provide pain relief and relieve tension.

Heat

You may have a hot water bottle at home and if you're suffering with muscle aches and pains, this low-tech approach can help you a great deal. Heat is soothing, and it's also healing, when applied correctly.

Heat opens up the blood vessels, increasing the blood supply to the affected area. This blood carries oxygen and nutrients to the painful area and also carries away cell waste material. Additionally, heat relaxes. It reduces muscle tension and can relieve painful spasms. These relaxant properties help you move more easily and increase your range of motion.

In addition to the hot water bottle, hot compresses that have been soaked in warm water can also give pain relief. When these cool to room temperature, they should be reheated. Other ways of delivering heat to painful areas include heating pads and commercial-grade gel packs.

STABS AND JABS

Don't get burned! Always wrap a hot water bottle, heating pad, or hot gel pack in a protective layer of toweling before applying it to your skin.

You can use heat packs for 10 to 15 minutes at a time several times a day.

Cold

Cold works the opposite way of heat. Instead of increasing the blood supply to the affected area, it slows it down. This helps to reduce inflammation and swelling, both sources of pain. It can also help control muscle spasms. Cold therapy is also called cryotherapy.

Cold compresses that have been soaked in cold water or cold gel packs can be applied to the skin where it's painful. As with hot packs, these should first be wrapped in an insulating towel layer to protect your skin.

Your therapist can also spray the painful area with fluoromethane, a refrigerant. It's related to the same chemicals that keep your freezer, air conditioner, and refrigerator cold.

For use at home, you can fill your hot water bottle with ice cubes or cold water from the tap. You can also use a package of frozen peas in a pinch. Replace the ice cubes or cold water when the bag or cold compress reaches room temperature and cook the peas for dinner.

You can use cold packs for 10 to 15 minutes at a time several times a day.

STABS AND JABS

Be careful! "Cold" or "ice" burns can be as painful as burns from a hot surface. Respect cold packs. Just because something's cold doesn't mean it can't bite back.

Paraffin Wax

Paraffin wax treatments are usually applied to hands and feet to improve circulation and provide pain relief. It's sometimes used to help alleviate the symptoms of arthritis. If you remember dipping your fingers into warm candle wax when you were a kid and peeling the cooled wax off in strips, then you have a general idea of how this treatment works. It's a little more involved, but the basic principles are the same.

If you're a bit nervous about molten wax on your skin, rest assured that's not the procedure. The wax is heated in a small vat until melted. Then you place your hand or your foot in the vat, coating the area that hurts. You then remove your hand or foot and allow the wax to set. You repeat this procedure several times until there are several layers of paraffin on your skin. The therapist then places a large mitten or towel over or around your foot or hand to hold in the heat. After the wax has thoroughly cooled, about 10 to 15 minutes, the mitten or towel is removed, and the wax peeled away. Your skin will feel cool.

POINTERS ON PAIN

Do not use a paraffin wax treatment if you are diabetic, have open sores or burns on your skin, or have any type of dermatitis.

Soft Tissue Mobilization

This is a bit different from the day spa variety massage, where you lie on the table and the massage therapist tends to your tired muscles while you breathe in the aroma from scented candles and relax to peaceful music.

Soft tissue mobilization administered by your physical therapist is designed to work on muscle tension and relieve muscle spasms by using pressure and friction. The goals go beyond relaxation, however, and focus on increasing flexibility and strength to help relieve your pain and getting the knotted muscle fibers to relax. Depending upon where your painful areas are, you'll either lie on a table or you'll sit in a chair during the therapy. There probably won't be any candles or any music.

Ultrasound

You're probably familiar with ultrasound as a diagnostic tool used to look at soft tissue injuries or to detect problems with various internal organs. It's also used for pain relief therapy, where its high-frequency sound waves are directed into painful muscles, generating mild heat, which is soothing and promotes improved circulation that helps reduce inflammation.

The same type of probe that's used in diagnostic ultrasound is used in physical therapy. The therapist first applies gel to the skin surface. This gel allows the probe to slide across the skin without creating friction or irritation. Then the probe is positioned over the painful area and moved in slow circles as the sound waves are dispatched to that site.

> **POINTERS ON PAIN**
>
> Ultrasound treatments are not recommended for pregnant women or for anyone with a metal implant.

TENS

TENS stands for Transcutaneous Electrical Nerve Stimulation. It's often used after the active portion of therapy to relax muscles, block pain signals from reaching the brain, and promote *endorphin* production. Small electrical currents are generated from the TENS machine and are delivered to painful areas via electrodes taped to your skin.

> **DEFINITION**
>
> **Endorphins** are the body's "feel good" hormones. They're produced during periods of intense exercise and result in what's commonly known as the "runner's high."

These electrodes may be placed on the skin right at the painful spot or along different locations on the nerve pathways. The procedure doesn't hurt. It does produce a tingling sensation, which is not unpleasant.

EMS

EMS, or Electrical Muscle Stimulation, is similar to TENS, although the electrodes placed on the skin are designed to deliver electrical impulses in a high enough dosage to cause the muscles to contract. The purpose of the procedure is to increase muscle strength by taking the muscles through a series of contractions and releases. It's like automatic reps!

EMS can increase circulation and improve muscle tone and strength, and that results in increased range of motion and greater flexibility.

Active Therapy

As you begin active therapy, your therapist may help you learn the proper positions by moving your body in the desired way. This is called active-assistive exercise, and as you get stronger, his role will decrease and yours will increase.

Starting with day one, take notes and ask questions. Your goal is to do these activities at home, so get all the information you need to be able to accomplish this. Most practices will have handouts for you, which give accurate and detailed instructions for each movement or exercise you'll be doing. Read these handouts when you're given them and be sure you understand exactly what they say. Have your therapist walk you through each exercise until you thoroughly understand what you're supposed to do, before you leave for home.

Stretching

Warm-ups are essential. Stretching before your major exercise segment will increase blood flow to your muscles, ligaments, and tendons and reduce your chance of injury to them. "Feed them before you use them" is your new mantra.

Stretch until you feel a slight pulling, but don't overstretch. Overstretching will put your muscles in a protective mode, and they'll fight you to prevent injury to themselves. Treat them with some tender respect, and they'll cooperate.

POINTERS ON PAIN

Don't "bounce" when you're doing your stretching warm-ups. Slow, even stretches are more effective, and you won't run the risk of tearing a muscle or straining a ligament.

Watch your posture as you're stretching. Keep your back straight! Your therapist will provide you with a list of stretching exercises tailored specifically to your needs.

Cool-downs are as important as warm-ups. Stretching after your exercises will help your muscles slow down and relax and eliminate any excess *lactic acid* that's built up there.

DEFINITION

Lactic acid is produced in your muscles during strenuous exercise, as blood sugar (glucose) is metabolized.

When you first begin your therapy program, your muscles will tire easily. As you increase your fitness level, you'll see dramatic results in pain relief, but you can't rush the process. It can take several weeks to achieve a better level of fitness.

Range-of-Motion Exercises

Each of your body's joints has a range of motion. It can extend (called extension) and flex (called flexion). Injury or a medical condition such as arthritis can decrease your joints' range of motion. If your joints are painful when you move them, you tend to move them less. This decreases their range of motion over time and getting them to function normally again can take time and effort.

There's no simple way around this. To increase your range of motion once it's been compromised, you'll need to move that joint beyond the point it becomes painful. Then you release. There should be no residual pain after you've done this exercise. Residual pain is pain that continues after you've let the joint relax.

As you continue these exercises, your range of motion will increase, and the pain will decrease. It is important to follow your therapist's instructions carefully to get the correct results.

Strengthening Exercises

Strengthening exercises work by putting muscles under resistance. In fact, strengthening exercises are also called resistance exercises. At each session, you'll increase the amount of resistance you apply by using weights or bands. As your muscles get stronger, they become less painful.

There are two types of strengthening exercises: isometric and isotonic. In isometric exercise (also called static strength training), you push against something without changing the length of the muscle or moving a joint.

For example, if you have muscle spasms in your lower back, here's an exercise to help you relieve them:

1. Lie on your back with your knees flexed.

2. Support your calves and feet with pillows.

3. Then push your lower back against the floor.

4. Hold this position for 10 seconds and then relax.

Gradually, you'll be able to increase your repetitions and strengthen your lower back muscles, preventing spasms and the pain they cause.

Strengthening your abdominal muscles will also help you decrease overall back pain. The main muscles you want to target here are the transverse abdominus muscle and the rectus abdominis. Losing the extra belly fat will also help you relieve low back pain, so get serious about your exercises, eat nutritious meals, and you'll be feeling better soon.

Low-Impact Aerobics

These exercises build endurance and combat fatigue, a common cause of low back pain. Your physical therapist will have a treadmill, an elliptical, stationary bicycles, and various other types of aerobic equipment for you to use during your therapy session.

When you're no longer going to therapy, the easiest form of low-impact aerobic exercise is walking. Swimming is also easy on your joints, if you've got access to a pool.

Hydrotherapy

Hydrotherapy means "water therapy," and it can be used as passive therapy and as a medium in which active therapy can be performed. Hydrotherapy venues cover a broad spectrum, ranging from hot tubs to swimming pools. The water can be cool, warm, or hot, depending upon the vehicle of delivery. Cool water is used for reducing inflammation; warm and hot water increase blood flow to inflamed areas, bringing oxygen and nutrients to promote healing.

Whirlpools or Jacuzzis have jets that shoot out streams of warm water that you can direct to the points on your body that hurt. Their pulsing action works like a massage to relieve muscle pain.

At home, if you don't have a Jacuzzi, you can invest in a showerhead that has different settings that can deliver pulsating shots of water to the parts that hurt. The only drawback to a shower massage is getting a good angle while not slipping on the wet tiles.

About Occupational Therapy

Occupational therapists can give you the tools to help you better manage your own self-care with the least amount of pain. With your particular medical condition in mind, occupational therapy can mean teaching you the most efficient way to bathe, dress, and perform household chores. It can also mean modifying your work environment and the way you get to work, to help you manage pain more efficiently.

SPEAKING OF PAIN

Most states regulate occupational therapy practice. Their professional organization is the American Occupational Therapy Association.

As with physical therapy, your insurance company may cover some or all of the costs of your occupational therapy. (See "Insurance Coverage" earlier in this chapter.)

Your life is about more than work and chores, however. Your occupational therapist can show you how to "get back in the game," so you can enjoy your hobbies and other recreational activities. If you have arthritis, this may mean helping you protect painful joints by fitting you with an orthotic device, such as a splint or brace to be worn while engaged in a specific activity that may cause you joint pain.

Your First Appointment

At your first appointment, you'll sit down with your occupational therapist and review your medical history, the specific pain issues you have, and your goals for managing that pain.

You'll most likely go through your day's schedule with the therapist and discuss which of the activities increase your pain. Your therapy will then focus on showing you how to perform these activities in a more comfortable manner.

Assistive Devices

Your occupational therapist has catalogues filled with labor-saving devices that can be ordered to make your life much easier and less painful. From reach extenders that allow you to retrieve items on the top shelf without straining your muscles to push-button can openers, the list of items is extensive.

Tricks of the Trade

There is an easy way and a hard way to do almost anything, and your occupational therapist is your resource for finding out the easiest way. Until someone points out the obvious, it's not all that obvious.

For example, if you love to garden but can't kneel on the ground without aggravating your knees, your occupational therapist will help you brainstorm options—everything from using raised beds for growing flowers and vegetables to searching out garden tools designed with extra-wide grips that are easier on arthritic hands.

The operative word is "ergonomic," and it's one word your occupational therapist lives by. It's all about proper body mechanics and developing good habits. As far as your body is concerned, this means using the largest body surface you can for the task at hand. Big muscle groups are stronger than small groups.

With physical and occupational therapy to guide you, you can live more pain-free. That's a good goal to strive for!

The Least You Need to Know

- Physical therapy can help you achieve greater functionality and also keep pain from getting worse.
- Strengthening your muscles can relieve joint pain.
- Improving your flexibility can relieve muscle spasms and prevent low back pain.
- Resistance exercises build muscle strength and help relieve and prevent pain.
- Occupational therapy can help you perform daily tasks more efficiently and with less pain.
- Assistive devices can take the strain off sore muscles.

Expanding Your Pain Relief Options

In This Chapter

- Harnessing the power of the mind-body connection
- What Eastern medicine has to offer
- The healing power of touch
- Nature's medicines

Taking the broad view can be immensely helpful in your quest for pain relief. In addition to medications and physical therapy, you have additional resources at your command. These approaches to treatment used to be labeled "alternative." Today, however, many of them are seen as good adjuncts to traditional methods of pain management. Many of them are focused on self-empowerment, and others rely on traditional practices of Eastern medicine.

Self-Empowerment Strategies

Pain is like an ink spot on a blotter. It spreads until it comes into contact with something that can stop it. Many times this something is the edge of the blotter. With pain, that *something* can be as simple as coming to the decision that you've reached the end of your patience and you're not going to let pain control your life any longer.

You can empower yourself in many ways, and you don't have to restrict yourself to just one or even a few options. Explore, expand, and enrich your life, while you're looking for the right combination of strategies and practices that will give you lasting relief from pain. An added benefit is that many of these self-empowerment strategies don't cost a penny and require no special equipment.

Learning to Cope

It's important to keep in mind that today's common remedies were once only possibilities. Medical advances happen quickly, and just because no answers are available for you today doesn't mean they won't be coming along in the near future. Every day medical science makes breakthroughs. Today or tomorrow may bring the breakthrough you're waiting for.

If you find, despite all your efforts at diagnosis, that a cause for your pain simply can't be found, what do you do? You know the pain is real. You know that it has a profound negative impact on your quality of life. You also know that you're going to have to find a way to cope.

Positive Thinking

Are you a glass-half-empty or a glass-half-full person? If you fit into the former category, you're generally looking at situations from a worst-case scenario. If you fit into the latter category, you're an optimist, always looking on the brighter side. Most of us are realists, understanding that life has ups and downs, good points and bad ones.

Pain is one of those bad points. Changing your focus means thinking about pain differently. Instead of dwelling on how much you hurt, start thinking about the parts of you that are working just fine.

We have control over really very little in life, but if we can't control the situation, we can control our response to it, whatever the situation may be. If we feel powerless in the face of pain, that causes the pain to feel worse. It takes control.

A tiny paper cut can change your whole mood. For a minute or two it's all you can think about. No wonder, then, that bigger and chronic pain can have such a pervasive effect. Fortunately, you can treat these extremes of the pain spectrum with the same technique: daily *affirmations*.

> **DEFINITION**
>
> **Affirmations** are positive self-talk. They're designed to increase your self-esteem, promote a sense of well-being, and give you control over negative situations.

Each day you have many opportunities to reinforce positive thoughts about your pain management protocol. For example, if you're exercising regularly and eating a healthy diet, turn this fact into an affirmation. When pain bothers you, say, "Every day I am making my body stronger and more resistant to pain."

If you're taking your medications as directed, you can turn this into an affirmation as well. "My medication is going to the source of my pain, and I will be helping my body."

Continue to look for opportunities to turn healthy practices into affirmations. Repeat them often until they become part of you and use them to manage your pain.

POINTERS ON PAIN

Whatever your medical condition, there is a support group made up of people just like you, sharing information and encouraging each other. Ask your physician, check with your local hospital, or go online to find the group you're looking for.

Meditation

If you haven't tried meditation as a pain management technique because you thought it was too complicated, you'll be relieved to learn that meditation is simply the act of clearing your mind of distracting thoughts. The goal of meditation is a peaceful mind and a calm spirit, and you achieve this by controlling your breathing, practicing visualization, and relaxing your body.

When you're in pain, your breathing tends to be rapid and shallow. Slowing down your breathing and taking deeper, measured breaths allows your body to take in more oxygen that it needs to heal damaged tissues. The mind can focus on only one thing at a time. When you're focused on your breathing, you're not focused on your pain. It's really that simple.

Meditation requires that you free your mind of disturbing thoughts. You do this by focusing your energy on something neutral, such as a sound or a pleasant scene. The principle is the same as with your breathing. Your mind focuses on this one thing to the exclusion of everything else, and that includes your pain.

With practice, meditation becomes easier, your body relaxes more, and your stress level decreases. The happy result is that your pain becomes manageable.

Humor and Laughter

This is a cause-and-effect relationship. Laughter has been scientifically proven to reduce stress, promote endorphin release, and decrease sensations of pain. Does this mean that pain is funny? Not in the least, but you can find humor in just about any situation, and once you do, that situation loses its power to control you. Humor is finding a bit of the absurd in whatever life tosses at you. Laughter is a response to that humor. It's not a coincidence that humor and laughter can be found in the most difficult of circumstances. It's nature's way of helping us cope. From gentle ribbing to those tired old jokes that are true groaners, humor can be good pain relief.

Laughter all by itself can also be beneficial in relieving pain. It may seem odd, but laughter yoga has become increasingly widespread and popular. Begun by yoga practitioner Dr. Madan Kataria from Mumbai, India, laughter yoga was first introduced in 1995. The practice combines yoga breathing and laughter.

The human body cannot distinguish between laughter generated as a response to something humorous and laughter initiated without such a stimulus. Using this knowledge, Dr. Kataria's laughter yoga has resulted in laughter clubs springing up worldwide. They are simply a place to go to practice yogic breathing and laughter. If you're interested in learning more, go to www.laughteryoga.org.

> **POINTERS ON PAIN**
>
> Self-medicating with alcohol is never a good idea. Alcohol consumption can interfere with your sleep, and your body needs sleep to heal.

Cognitive Behavioral Therapy (CBT)

The principle behind Cognitive Behavioral Therapy (CBT) is that your thoughts control your feelings. By learning how to control your thoughts, you can control the way you feel, and if you're in pain, this means you can change the way you experience pain.

Your physician can refer you to a *psychotherapist* to learn how to put CBT to work to manage your pain.

> **DEFINITION**
>
> A **psychotherapist** is a licensed mental health professional, such as a psychiatrist, psychologist, or counselor, who can work with you to resolve issues that negatively affect your quality of life.

Biofeedback

You may think that your blood pressure and brain wave activity are not something you have much control over, and that used to be the accepted medical thinking. We now know, however, that it's possible to harness the power of the mind to control certain body functions of the autonomic nervous system that previously were thought to be involuntary.

Since stress intensifies the pain experience, it makes sense that anything that reduces stress will also help relieve pain. Biofeedback can do this. Your physician can refer you to a clinic where you will learn how to use biofeedback as a pain-management technique.

There are many ways to do biofeedback. One method requires a technician to attach electrodes to your skin. These electrodes transmit information either as a tone, as lines moving across a grid on a computer screen, or as different levels of brightness on a visual meter.

Next the technician leads you through different mental exercises, and your responses show up as data. Those responses that show up as positive data can be reinforced. Essentially, you learn how to control your body's autonomic nervous system. You can then relax your muscles, decrease stress, and manage your pain.

Traditional Eastern Practices

The philosophy behind *Eastern medicine* is that the mind, the body, and the spirit are all one. That belief has created a holistic system of healing. In recent years, Western medicine has come to embrace certain aspects of this holistic philosophy. Today, Complementary and Alternative Therapy (CAT) is considered a valuable addition to the healing arts of Western medicine.

DEFINITION

Eastern medicine refers to a variety of healing practices and products that originated in the Orient, from India to China and other countries in this area. Eastern medicine developed its own traditions, and its philosophy centers on restoring balance.

Acupuncture

Acupuncture originated more than 2,000 years ago and has been a staple of Chinese medicine since that time. It operates from the belief that energy, called *qi*, flows through the body along certain channels. When the *qi* gets blocked, illness and pain result. Acupuncture works to restore the natural flow of the body's *qi*.

The term acupuncture means "prickling needle," and that's exactly what happens during an acupuncture treatment. The acupuncturist will first discuss the nature of your pain with you and then will insert tiny needles in your skin along specific pathways or meridians. This pattern of placement is specific to your problem. Once the pattern is complete, the needles will remain in place for about half an hour. You'll rest quietly during this time. Then the acupuncturist removes the needles, and you're free to go on your way.

> **SPEAKING OF PAIN**
>
> Acupuncture needles are either disposable or are used only once before they're autoclaved to sterilize them so there is no risk of transmitting disease with them.

It's believed that the needles stimulate your body's production of endorphins, the "feel good" hormones. Your physician may refer you to a licensed acupuncturist, or she may be an acupuncturist herself. More and more physicians are these days.

Your insurance carrier may pay part or all of the cost of an acupuncture treatment and may require preauthorization, so check with them before you schedule your appointment.

Yoga

The practice of yoga originated in the Indus Valley thousands of years ago and is another Eastern practice that centers on restoring balance to the body by healing the mind-body-spirit connection. Instead of *qi*, however, yoga focuses on *prana*, which is the body's life force. The goal is to seek understanding of life's purpose and union with the universal consciousness.

Chronic pain is a thief. It robs you of a sense of control over your body, but yoga is a discipline that can return that feeling of control to you and help you manage chronic pain. You may worry that the postures you've seen in pictures will hurt and decide that yoga isn't for you. But there is a great deal more involved than just postures. Yoga combines aspects of breathing, meditation, and those precise postures to relieve stress and anxiety—both of which make the pain experience worse.

Check with your physician before you begin to study yoga. When you have the go-ahead, begin slowly and build your strength over time. Yoga sessions begin with gentle stretching exercises designed to build flexibility. Increasing your flexibility can be extremely helpful if you have arthritis pain.

You can find beginning yoga classes through your local hospital or community center, as well as through the YMCA or YWCA. And remember, there are many different types of yoga. Everything from sivananda yoga, to hatha yoga, to ashtanga yoga, to iyengar yoga require you to focus on different elements from breathing, stretching, strengthening, and meditating. Do some research and find a good fit for you.

Tai Chi

Tai chi originated in China as one of the martial arts. Its original use was as a form of self-defense, and you can tap into this aspect of it to defend your body from the effects of chronic pain. Like yoga, tai chi is designed to increase flexibility. Unlike yoga, tai chi's movements are orchestrated from a standing position.

Watching people going through their tai chi movements is something similar to watching a ballet. Each dancer is focused on his or her routine and it's a graceful performance to observe.

Tai chi has more than 100 different movements, and after you've selected the ones that you're comfortable doing and which help you manage your pain, you'll practice them until one movement flows seamlessly into the next.

Community centers, your local hospital, senior centers, or your local YMCA or YWCA can direct you to a tai chi group in your area. Check out www.taichiforarthritis.com for additional information.

POINTERS ON PAIN

A *neti pot* is a traditional Indian method for dealing with sinus pain. Shaped like a miniature teapot, it is filled with a cleansing saline solution, and the spout is inserted into the nostril to deliver the solution, which shrinks nasal membranes and helps promote drainage.

Hands-On Therapy

Touch is one of the five senses, and it's much more involved than being just a vehicle for giving us information about our world. In a very real sense, touch connects us to our world more than any other of the senses. Without touch, babies fail to thrive. Without touch, we feel isolated and alone. Touch is essential for our well-being, and therapeutic touch can help manage chronic pain.

Massage

Therapeutic massage involves the manipulation of the body's muscles and connective tissues with the purpose of increasing blood flow and promoting better circulation. The goal of massage is to reduce stress, tension, and anxiety and provide relief from chronic pain.

POINTERS ON PAIN

Studies have confirmed the benefits of massage in managing arthritis pain, low back pain, and pain associated with pregnancy.

If your physician has referred you to physical therapy, massage may be part of your therapy session. Your insurance carrier may cover part or all of the expense of massage therapy, so be sure to check before you schedule your appointment.

Chiropractic

Chiropractic is the most frequently used form of complementary and alternative medicine. It involves the manipulation or adjustment of joints. Chiropractors are not medical doctors, even though they use the initials D.C. (Doctor of Chiropractic) after their names.

Chiropractic was invented by an Iowa grocer by the name of David Palmer. He was looking for a way to cure disease without using drugs or other medications and decided that manipulation was the way to go. If you visit a chiropractor, it's most likely that he or she is a graduate of the Palmer method. Chiropractors must have a minimum of two years of college and four years in a school of chiropractic in order to be licensed.

Although not recommended for individuals with rheumatoid arthritis, many people do find that chiropractic affords pain relief for osteoarthritis and other joint conditions. Check with your doctor before deciding to use a chiropractor to be sure it's safe for your particular pain issues.

Herbs and Supplements

Using plants to relieve pain goes back to the dawn of time, when the first seeker chewed on a piece of willow bark and found that it eased the pain of a toothache or perhaps a sore muscle. It was a discovery that changed the world, and we still reap the benefits of it today. The chemical found in willow bark, salicylic acid, became the basis for aspirin, the world's most commonly used drug for pain.

Aspirin has been studied extensively for its therapeutic properties. Its manufacture and quality are assured because it is regulated through the U.S. Food and Drug Administration (FDA). This is not the case, however, with dietary supplements and herbs. They do not fall under the jurisdiction of the FDA, and this fact should be food for thought before you make the decision to expand your pain relief options through the use of these products.

Botanicals

Botanicals are products manufactured from plants or plant parts. You may see them labeled as herbal products, phytomedicines (*phyto* being the Latin word for "plant"), or botanicals. Some botanicals fall under the classification of food products, and as such can be regulated by the FDA. Some botanicals are outside this definition, and as a consequence are not regulated by the FDA.

 STABS AND JABS

Don't be confused by the term "all natural." Just because something comes from nature doesn't mean it's benign. Some natural substances are poisons!

Many botanicals with pain-relieving properties are familiar ingredients in cooking. Turmeric and ginger, for example, have shown some merit in relieving the symptoms of osteoarthritis.

Other common garden plants, such as feverfew, have been used to treat the pain of migraine headaches.

Supplements

Dietary supplements, specifically glucosamine and chondroitin, have been widely touted as treatments for relieving the pain of osteoarthritis as well as for their benefit in regenerating cartilage.

Studies into the beneficial effects of these two supplements have produced conflicting results. Some studies say the supplements work, and others found no benefit to be derived from either of them.

If you decide to give glucosamine and chondroitin a try, remember that dietary supplements are not regulated by the FDA. That means you have no guarantee as to the purity or the content of the capsules you buy.

STABS AND JABS

If you have allergies to shellfish, avoid both glucosamine and chondroitin. They are made from shells of shellfish and shark cartilage, respectively.

The Least You Need to Know

- When a cure isn't possible, learning to manage pain can help you live life to the fullest.
- Humor and laughter have been scientifically proven to relieve pain.
- Many practices taken from Eastern medicine, such as acupuncture, yoga, and tai chi, can help relieve pain and increase functionality.
- Herbal products and dietary supplements are not regulated by the FDA and should be used with caution and under your doctor's supervision.

Surgery

In This Chapter

- Relief for sinus pain
- Joint replacements
- Repairing or removing damaged organs
- Preparing yourself for surgery

Many types of pain respond to rest, medication, and physical therapy. There are times, however, when surgery is a reasonable course of action. Surgery is a decision you will make after discussing the pros and cons with your surgeon. Some types of surgery have high rates of success, while others may provide only temporary relief. In this chapter, we'll cover some common types of surgery designed to relieve pain.

Sinus Surgery

Repeated sinus infections and sinus headaches may lead you to the decision that surgery is the only way you're going to get relief. Endoscopic sinus surgery enlarges the openings that allow the sinuses to drain, restoring the normal drainage pattern. With drainage operating along more normal lines, sinus headache, congestion, and pain could be much improved.

The Procedure

Surgery is generally performed on an outpatient basis at a hospital or surgery center. You'll be given instructions concerning how to prepare for the surgery. You'll be asked to wash your face and not use any lotions, creams, or makeup on your face.

Your surgical team consists of the anesthesiologist, surgeon, nurse, and technician. You're definitely not on your own! After you're in the surgery room, the nurse or technician will start an intravenous (IV) drip and give you sedation prior to the anesthetic. The anesthetic will put you to sleep for the procedure, which can take up to several hours. The team carefully monitors all your vital signs while you're under the anesthetic. Your surgeon has already decided upon which procedure will work best for your condition.

One procedure is called *image guided endoscopic surgery,* and it's often used in cases of chronic sinusitis, when a patient has had previous sinus surgery, or when there are abnormalities in the structure of the sinuses. This surgery combines endoscopy with CT scans that show real-time movements using infrared signals.

> **SPEAKING OF PAIN**
>
> The American Academy of Otolaryngology reports that sinus surgery image guidance uses principles employed by the U.S. Armed Forces stealth bomb guidance system.

Another procedure to relieve the symptoms of chronic sinusitis is the Caldwell-Luc operation, which targets the maxillary sinus located beneath the eye. It is often used if there is a malignancy in the sinus cavity. The surgeon enters this sinus through the upper jaw and above the molars. Then he makes an opening to connect the sinus with the nose, allowing better drainage of the sinus cavity.

After the surgery, an absorbent packing is usually inserted into your nostrils to absorb any post-op bleeding. These packs will be removed at the doctor's office during your follow-up visit. You'll stay in recovery until you're fully awake and ready to go home.

Your Part

You'll be given instructions on what to do when you get home. Keeping your head elevated above your heart will help reduce any post-op swelling. Your surgeon will prescribe antibiotics to help prevent any infection and pain medications to get you through the initial post-operative discomfort.

After the nasal packing is removed, you'll begin using a saline nasal spray to keep the mucous membranes soft and prevent crusts from forming. Recovery may take up to a few weeks; during this time, you should refrain from strenuous activities. You should also avoid taking aspirin or any medications that contain aspirin during the recovery period, as these medications may cause the bleeding to continue. If you need pain medication, acetaminophen is considered safe to use.

 STABS AND JABS

Go easy on brushing your teeth until you have healed. Vigorous brushing irritates tender tissues.

The Tally Sheet

In most cases, sinus surgery is effective in achieving its objective, which is widening the drainage system. Overall success rates range from 75 to 95 percent improvement in symptoms. However, the surgery doesn't always provide a permanent fix to the problem. Endoscopic procedures generally entail fewer risks than open surgery, but endoscopic sinus surgery does come with some risks. These risks can include:

- General risks associated with anesthesia
- Post-operative bleeding in the nose
- Infection and formation of scar tissue in the nose
- Damage to facial nerves
- Leakage of spinal fluid (in about 2 percent of surgeries)
- Blindness (rare) due to damage of the optic nerve during surgery

Sinus surgery may be the answer to your pain, but surgery should always be the last option.

Carpal Tunnel Surgery

Carpal tunnel surgery is performed to take pressure off the median nerve in the wrist. It's done using a local anesthetic on an outpatient basis. There are two approaches to carpal tunnel surgery: open release surgery (the traditional method) and endoscopic surgery (the newer method).

The Procedure

In open release surgery, your surgeon will make an incision about 2 inches long in the wrist and then cut the carpal ligament. This will widen the carpal tunnel. In the endoscopic approach, the surgeon will make one small incision in your palm and one in your wrist. These incisions are only about ½ inch long, but they're big enough to allow the endoscope to enter and cut the ligament.

Recovery from the endoscopic procedure is usually quicker than the open release surgery because less area is involved and less tissue needs to heal.

Your Part

Since this is usually done on an outpatient basis, you'll generally be able to go home shortly after the procedure has been completed. Your surgeon may prescribe a non-steroidal anti-inflammatory drug (NSAID) to take until any swelling has subsided. Your physician may refer you to a physical therapist after your surgery to regain strength and function in the wrist.

The Tally Sheet

Results are generally good, with more people reporting a higher success rate with the endoscopic procedure as opposed to open release. Risks can include damage to the median nerve and infection.

Joint Replacement Surgery

When osteoarthritis or rheumatoid arthritis has damaged a joint to the point that it's no longer functional and is a source of constant pain, surgery to replace that joint is an option many people pursue. The procedure to replace a joint is called *arthroplasty*. There are two approaches to joint replacement.

The Procedure

The first option is called *joint resection*. For this procedure the surgeon goes into the troublesome joint and removes part of the bone. Scar tissue forms. This enlargement of the joint space results in increased range of motion and also relieves pain.

The second option is called *joint replacement*. For this procedure the surgeon replaces the diseased cartilage and bone with a prosthetic one.

These procedures are performed in a hospital or surgery center where you are an in-patient. You'll receive a general anesthetic so you'll be asleep for the procedure. After the surgery, you'll generally remain in the hospital for a few days, but your physical therapy will begin almost immediately after you're out of recovery and back in your room. It usually takes at least six weeks of physical therapy and daily exercising to strengthen the ligaments and rejuvenate the muscles that support the joint that's undergone surgery.

> **SPEAKING OF PAIN**
>
> A replacement joint has an average life span of 7 to 10 years before it needs to be replaced.

If your problem is just on one side of the joint, another option, called *osteotomy*, can realign the bones to take stress off the part of the joint that's affected and transfer that stress to the healthy side. This procedure is usually indicated in a knee joint that angles inward.

When this procedure is performed on a hip joint, the surgeon cuts the bones in the joint, repositions them, and then stabilizes them in the new position.

Osteotomy is done under general anesthesia. Complete recovery may take several months. The benefit of this surgery is that it can postpone a total joint replacement by up to 10 years.

Your Part

Your preparation for surgery begins weeks before you actually enter the hospital. Statistics prove that the better shape you're in before surgery, the faster your recovery will be, and the more successful the results.

The American Academy of Orthopaedic Surgeons has provided specific recommendations for getting your body ready for surgery. These include quitting smoking (or at least cutting down). Smoking has many negative effects on your body, including slowing down the healing process.

Exercise is essential to a good outcome. Find out now what your post-operative physical therapy program will entail and get an early start on following this routine now to the best of your ability. This will make it easier to get with the program after your joint replacement.

For knee or hip replacements, work on strengthening your upper arms and chest muscles. If you'll be using crutches or a walker, you'll be glad your upper body is able to carry the weight. Following the post-operative therapy plan is essential to a successful result.

The Tally Sheet

Joint replacement surgeries are becoming common, as an aging population looks for viable ways to keep active. In 2003 (the last year for which statistics are available), the Centers for Disease Control and Prevention reported that more than 638,000 hip or knee replacement surgeries were done. The numbers are expected to increase each year.

Risks of these surgeries include the risks associated with all surgeries: reaction to anesthesia, possibility of blood clots, and infection. Joints can loosen or wear out and require additional surgery to replace them. This surgery is called *revision total joint replacement*, and it comes with increased risks.

 SPEAKING OF PAIN

The most serious risk associated with joint replacement surgery is a 1 percent chance of death within three months after the first surgery and a 2.6 percent risk of death after a second surgery.

Hysterectomy

A hysterectomy is a surgical procedure to remove the uterus. There are different degrees of hysterectomy. In a total hysterectomy, the ovaries and the cervix are removed along with the uterus. A radical hysterectomy may be indicated in the presence of certain kinds of cancer. This procedure, in addition to removing the uterus, cervix, and ovaries, also removes tissue along both sides of the cervix and the upper portion of the vagina.

The Procedure

In addition to the traditional abdominal method, modern technologies have resulted in new surgical techniques for hysterectomies. Different surgical approaches are indicated in different situations. The most common procedures include the following:

- **Abdominal**—This is the original method for performing a hysterectomy. The surgeon makes an incision across the lower part of the abdomen, usually just above the pubic bone. In some cases the incision may be vertical instead of horizontal. In any case, it's about 5 to 7 inches in length.

- **Vaginal**—The surgeon makes a small incision in the vagina and uses an endoscopic procedure to remove the uterus through this incision.

- **Laparascopic**—The surgeon makes two or three small incisions in your abdomen and uses the laparascope to cut the uterus into sections small enough to be removed through these incisions.

Generally, recovery from a vaginal or laparascopic hysterectomy is quicker and easier than from an abdominal one. This is because in an abdominal hysterectomy, the area involved is bigger, the incision is larger, and the muscles must heal.

POINTERS ON PAIN

A patient who undergoes a total hysterectomy will experience immediate onset of menopause because the organs responsible for menstruation will have been removed. Talk with your doctor about the pros and cons of estrogen replacement therapy.

After surgery, you'll be moved to recovery until you are awake and ready to go back to your room. You'll have an IV that administers pain medication and fluids, and you may also have a catheter in your bladder to assist in elimination of urine. The catheter generally is removed the day after surgery.

You'll be encouraged to use the bathroom as soon as possible and to get up and move about. You'll be discharged usually within two to three days. It can take several weeks to heal after a hysterectomy, and it's important not to try to speed up the process by doing more than you should. Rest is essential, along with mild activity to speed healing.

You should refrain from sexual intercourse until you are fully healed from the surgery. This will take from six to eight weeks. Engaging in sexual relations before you are fully healed will be painful.

Your Part

Remember, a hysterectomy is major surgery, regardless of the size of the incision. While you are healing, it's important to balance rest with exercise, but avoid lifting heavy objects. Follow your doctor's instructions and you'll heal quickly.

The Tally Sheet

Many women experience few if any lingering aftereffects from the surgery, and freedom from pain is often cited as the principal benefit. Risks can include all those associated with any surgery, including the possibility of infection, blood clot, or reaction to anesthesia.

Back Surgeries

Back pain can be stubborn to treat. Medications and physical therapy aren't always effective in relieving the pain. You may be considering surgery as a once-and-for-all fix, but surgery isn't always effective in solving the pain problem. There are some instances, though, when surgery does make sense. Back surgery is performed under anesthesia. In most cases, that means a general anesthetic. This section covers some of the more common back surgeries and weighs the pros and cons of each.

Discectomy

A discectomy is a procedure to remove troublesome discs, and is performed when a disc has ruptured (herniated) and is pressing on the spinal cord or nerve roots. A radiculopathy (or a pinched nerve) is the most common reason for performing a discectomy.

The Procedure

All or just a portion of the disc may be removed. Sometimes the surgeon will perform a laminectomy (see the preceding section) to be able to work more easily in the area.

Depending on the amount of disc material that has been removed, the two vertebrae may or may not be fused as well.

POINTERS ON PAIN

A discectomy may be performed endoscopically or as open surgery. Speak with your surgeon to see which is the best choice for your problem.

Your Part

If there are no complications, you'll usually be able to go home the following day. You'll be given instructions to avoid lifting, bending, or twisting during the healing process. Physical therapy is generally recommended.

The Tally Sheet

Discectomy has been shown to be of substantial benefit to people with severe pain from herniated disks. Risks include all those associated with any surgery, including reaction to anesthetic, infection at the surgical site, and blood clots. Additionally, there is the possibility of nerve damage at the site.

Laminectomy

This procedure, called a laminectomy, involves removing parts of the vertebrae. It is generally performed on the lumbar spine (lower spine), most often to relieve the pain and dysfunction from spinal stenosis.

The Procedure

The surgeon makes an incision along the midline of your back and removes a small part of the vertebrae over the nerve root. Sometimes a portion of the disc is also excised. The goal is to give the nerve more room so that it's not under constant pressure.

Your Part

The hospital stay for a laminectomy is generally short, from one to three days. You'll be on your feet and walking very quickly after this procedure but won't be allowed to do any lifting, twisting, or bending for the duration of the healing process, which takes about six weeks.

The Tally Sheet

Success rates range from 70 to 80 percent, with most people able to function more easily and with reduced pain after surgery.

X-STOP Surgery

X-STOP surgery is a newer procedure done to relieve low back and leg pain associated with spinal stenosis.

The Procedure

Your surgeon will implant a titanium device, called the X-STOP, in your back at the place where the nerves are being compressed.

DEFINITION

X-STOP stands for Interspinous Process Decompression System. The device was approved by the FDA in 2005.

In some cases, this procedure may be used instead of laminectomy. The device is designed to give you more space in the vertebral canal to stop aggravating the nerves. It does permit you to move forward and rotate your lower back with minimal limitations.

If your surgeon agrees that you are a candidate for X-STOP surgery, the procedure will most likely be done on an outpatient basis. It's a shorter procedure than a laminectomy, and you'll be in recovery within the hour. You'll usually be able to go home the same day, although your surgeon may have you stay in the hospital for a day or so to be sure there are no complications.

Your Part

You'll receive instructions to begin walking right away. Walking helps your blood flow more effectively, bringing oxygen and other nutrients to the surgical site, promoting healing. Avoid bending, lifting, twisting, and other activities that stress your back during the healing process.

POINTERS ON PAIN

Spinal decompression surgery is a general term that includes various procedures, including laminectomy and discectomy, among others. The purpose is to relieve pressure on nerves associated with the spinal cord.

The Tally Sheet

Risks for X-STOP surgery include all those associated with any surgery, including infection at the surgical site, blood clots, and reaction to the anesthetic. Additionally, damage to blood vessels, pneumonia, heart attack, stroke, paralysis, or death are rare complications.

Benefits can include immediate pain relief. A two-year research study confirmed the benefit of X-STOP surgery in 50 percent of patients followed during the study period. Studies have not confirmed the lasting benefit of X-STOP surgery beyond that time frame.

Kyphoplasty

Compression fractures are often the result of osteoporosis and are frequently found among the elderly. As the bone deteriorates over time, gravity takes its toll, and this vertebra collapses onto the one beneath it. An endoscopic surgical procedure called kyphoplasty is used to repair the damage.

The Procedure

During this operation, the surgeon inserts a surgical instrument, called a bone tamp, with a balloon attached to it into the damaged portion of the vertebra. He then inflates the balloon until the normal position of the vertebra has been re-established. He fills the space inside the balloon with bone cement, removes the bone tamp, and closes the incision.

Your Part

After discharge from the hospital, you'll begin a program of physical therapy, designed to strengthen the muscles that support your spine and increase your flexibility and range of motion. You may be prescribed a back brace to wear for a specific period of time.

The Tally Sheet

Risks for kyphoplasty involve all risks associated with surgery, including infection, blood clots, nerve damage, paralysis, and reaction to anesthetic. Success rates for this procedure are good if the compression fracture being treated is not very old.

Arthrodesis

Arthrodesis is a procedure for fusing bones in the spine. It may be indicated if you've fractured one or more vertebrae in your spine, or if you have severe scoliosis. Fusing two or more of the vertebrae stabilizes them, which can relieve pain. In the case of scoliosis, the fusion straightens the curve to a better degree of functionality. Fusion is also done when discs have ruptured or have become so damaged that less invasive treatment isn't effective.

For this procedure, the surgeon inserts bone grafts in front, behind, around, or in between the injured vertebrae. As the body heals, these grafts grow into the vertebrae, joining them together. Before the incision is closed, metal plates, screws, or wires may be used to secure the graft while healing takes place.

Your Part

Arthrodesis is performed on an in-patient basis, and you'll remain in the hospital for a few days after the surgery to recover. During the recovery period after you're discharged, it's extremely important to follow your surgeon's instructions, and it can take a minimum of six weeks before the healing process is well underway. During this time, your physician may prescribe a back brace for you to wear. Walking, swimming, and riding a stationary bicycle are often parts of your physical therapy program after surgery.

The Tally Sheet

The effectiveness of arthrodesis for treating low back pain has not been proven. If surgery has been necessitated by presence of a tumor, trauma, or infection, it is important to understand the risks involved.

On the plus side, the spine should be more stable and in better alignment. Risks, however, include the possibility of blood clots (deep vein thrombosis), rejection of the graft, injury to the nerves, infection, and pain at the graft site.

Arthroscopy

You may be familiar with this surgical procedure. Often done on an outpatient basis, arthroscopy is frequently performed to remove damaged cartilage from the knee. The culprit here is usually osteoarthritis, although rheumatoid arthritis can also be involved.

Arthroscopy began as a diagnostic procedure, allowing the physician to see inside the joint prior to open surgery. Today, with advances in technology, arthroscopy can also be used as a medical procedure in its own right.

The Procedure

You'll be given either a general or a local anesthetic via regional blocks. In either case, an anesthesiologist or dedicated anesthesia staff will be present. Then your surgeon makes an incision over the joint. The arthroscope is inserted into the incision and a small camera attached to the instrument relays real-time pictures, which are displayed on a computer screen. These pictures help guide the surgeon's hand.

The surgeon injects water into the joint to expand it and allow enough room for the procedure to take place. The cartilage is removed and the incision is covered with a sterile dressing.

Your Part

You'll need to have someone drive you home after the procedure. Your rehabilitation program will begin almost immediately. Physical therapy will get you moving quickly and using your joint should be much less painful.

The Tally Sheet

Arthroscopy is a common procedure and has been quite effective in repairing torn cartilage or ligaments, thus reducing inflammation and relieving pain. Its benefits in treating knee osteoarthritis have been questioned and some research has indicated minimum to no benefit at all.

Risks include the possibility of infection at the surgical site, blood clots, and reaction to the anesthetic.

Heart Surgeries

According to the National Institutes of Health, more than half a million heart surgeries are performed in the United States each year, and many of these are done to correct problems caused by coronary artery disease. The most commonly performed heart surgery is coronary artery bypass grafting (CABG).

"Open heart surgery" was the traditional method of effecting repairs. This meant opening the chest wall by cutting through the breastbone and then retracting the muscles to get to the heart. A machine took over the heart and lung function for the patient, while the surgeon worked on the damaged heart. Once the surgery was complete, the machine was disconnected, and the heart restarted.

Today, new technology has made some significant changes in how heart surgery is done. Minimally invasive surgery that makes use of endoscopic techniques is becoming more common. In some cases, the heart-lung bypass machine is not needed, and in others, it is. It all depends upon the type of problem you have and what your surgeon recommends.

Angioplasty

This procedure, also referred to as balloon angioplasty, is used to improve blood flow in a coronary artery. The National Heart, Lung, and Blood Institute (part of the National Institutes of Health) reports that this surgery is performed more than a million times a year in the United States.

If you've had a heart attack or if you have atherosclerosis, which has caused plaque to build up on your arteries and reduced their ability to carry blood, your surgeon may decide that coronary angioplasty is the best way to treat your chest pain and other symptoms. It can save your life.

The Procedure

In simple terms, the surgeon inserts a catheter into an artery either in the groin area or in the armpit. A wire is threaded through the artery to the blockage. Then the surgeon slips a tube that carries a balloon over the wire; when the tube reaches the blockage, the surgeon inflates the balloon. This presses the accumulated plaque back against the wall of the artery.

The balloon may be inflated and deflated several times until the passage is sufficiently wide to allow blood to flow more easily through the artery. Then everything is withdrawn, and the procedure is finished. To see a visual depiction of this procedure, complete with narration, go to the following website: www.nhlbi.nih.gov/health/dci/Diseases/Angioplasty/Angioplasty_During.html.

After the surgery, you'll be moved to recovery, where your vital signs will be monitored. You'll need to lie still so that the blood vessels in your groin or arm have a chance to close up.

Your Part

You'll be able to go home in a day or two with medication to prevent blood clots and instructions as to how much activity is recommended during your recovery period.

Remember that angioplasty isn't a cure for coronary artery disease. It's up to you to make sure you give yourself the best possible prognosis. This means adopting healthy nutritional and lifestyle choices:

- If you smoke, quit.

- Manage your weight.

- Increase your physical activity as recommended by your physician.

- Take your prescribed medications to keep your blood pressure or cholesterol under control.

The Tally Sheet

Angioplasty is a common procedure. There is a small risk of serious complications, including bleeding from the blood vessel where the catheter was situated, allergic reaction to dye given during the procedure or kidney damage from the dye, irregular heart rhythm, damage to blood vessels from catheter placement, heart attack, rupturing of a plaque that migrates, and stroke.

Coronary Bypass Surgery

Just as a freeway can bypass downtown traffic congestion, bypass surgery reroutes the new blood vessel around the damaged point of the blocked artery. Your surgeon has a choice of several blood vessels to use during this surgery.

The Procedure

If the vein is taken from a leg, one end is grafted to the blocked coronary artery and the other is sewn to an opening that's made in the aorta. If the internal mammary artery in your chest is used, then one end remains attached where it is, and the other end is rerouted to your coronary artery. In some cases, an artery (the radial artery) in your wrist may be used.

> **SPEAKING OF PAIN**
>
> It is not uncommon to bypass more than one artery during coronary bypass surgery. Sometimes three or even four arteries are bypassed.

Heart surgery requires some time post-op in the hospital, so expect to spend anywhere from a few days to a week before being discharged. Immediately after surgery you'll be taken to intensive care, where all your vital signs will be monitored. You'll have drainage tubes (two to three) in your chest for a day or so. These allow fluid to drain out so that you don't develop edema, or swelling, around the surgery site.

Your Part

After you're fully awake, you'll be moved from the ICU to your room to continue your recovery. Before you're discharged, your physical therapy will already have begun. You'll be given instructions on what levels of activity are permitted and what kinds of exercise you need to do.

The Tally Sheet

Benefits of coronary bypass surgery include increased blood flow and reduced possibility of heart attack or stroke. Risks may include blood clots, infection, heart attack, or stroke during the procedure, or problems with heart rhythm. In some cases, postpericardiotomy syndrome can develop. This consists of a low-grade fever and chest pain and may last up to six months.

STABS AND JABS

Recovery from heart surgery takes time. Don't expect to bounce back overnight. It can take several months to start feeling the way you hope to feel.

General Recommendations for All Surgeries

Having surgery is not something any of us want to think about. Discuss any questions you have with your surgeon. Be sure you understand the goal of your surgery. Is it for pain control, or to make sure a particular condition doesn't get progressively worse? For example, lumbar stenosis surgery works best when patients have leg pain while walking or standing. Lumbar stenosis can help patients walk more, but it may not decrease their back pain.

All surgery entails some risk, and so in a very real sense, all surgery is major surgery. Follow your surgeon's instructions and be sure to ask questions if you have them.

To give yourself the best possible outcome, spend as much time on preparing for your recovery as you need to. When you return home, you're going to be tired, and you're not going to feel like getting your room, your kitchen, or your work site ready to accommodate you. The time to do this is before the surgery.

Preparing the Kitchen

Take inventory of your groceries. Shop beforehand and stock up on easy-to-prepare or frozen meals. When you're preparing your meals in the days prior to surgery, make enough to freeze portions for meals during your convalescence.

Organize your kitchen and pantry for convenience. Bring down anything you regularly use for cooking or serving that's up high or down low and find a place for it at counter level. Reaching, bending, and twisting are generally not allowed after many types of surgery.

> **STABS AND JABS**
>
> Prevent falls and trips by keeping your home clutter-free. If you have scatter rugs, be sure they have grip-tight pads under them. Better yet, take them up until you're steady on your feet again.

Preparing the Rest of the House

Most likely, your surgeon will want you to balance rest with mild activity to help you heal faster. Resting doesn't come easy to many of us, and you'll have a difficult time with this if you haven't thought ahead about what you'll need.

The American College of Orthopaedic Surgeons has some excellent suggestions for getting ready for your homecoming. One of these is to set up a "recovery center." Think of it as Mission Control. In fact, that's what they recommend. Put the remote control next to the chair where you'll be sitting when you're ready to watch television.

Have your phone within reach. If you have a cell phone, it's a good idea to keep it with you at all times, just in case you need emergency assistance. Other items they recommend include tissues, wastebasket, drinking water, a radio, your favorite reading materials, and definitely, your medications.

The Least You Need to Know

- Sinus surgery widens the sinus cavities to promote drainage and give pain relief.
- Joint replacement surgery can restore your mobility and provide dramatic relief from the pain of osteoarthritis.

- Heart surgery has its best success rate when it's coupled with positive lifestyle changes.
- Depending on the reason for your pain, a hysterectomy may involve removal of the uterus, as well as the ovaries and cervix.
- Prepare your home for surgery, just as you prepare yourself, and you'll have an easier homecoming.

Pain from Head to Toe

Pain can strike at any place in the body. Sometimes it comes on quickly and leaves soon. Other times it comes on gradually and persists over time. If you're experiencing pain, this part will help you understand what you're dealing with and give you helpful information on taking the best course of action to alleviate that pain. In Part 3, we'll take a look at pain from head to toe.

Chapter 10

It's All in Your Head

In This Chapter

- Distinguishing one type of headache from another
- Treating and preventing headaches
- Sinus pressure and pain
- Facial nerve pain
- Your mouth at night—pain at work

In this case, "It's all in your head" is not a rude dismissal of your symptoms but an affirmation. Headaches are probably our most annoying and occasionally frightening experiences with pain. In this chapter, we'll cover the basic forms headaches take and also explore the other areas in your head that can be sources of pain—your mouth, your sinus cavities, and your clenched jaw.

When to See the Doctor

Most headaches are not critical emergencies, but some are. You should call 911 if:

- You are having "the worst headache of your life"
- Your headache came on as abruptly as if someone flipped on a light switch
- Lying down increases the severity of your headache
- You are having problems with your balance, speech, or vision that you've never experienced with a headache before
- Your headache began after a recent fall or injury to the head

Any of these symptoms may be due to stroke, bleeding in the brain, or another potentially life-threatening condition. Other serious symptoms that you shouldn't ignore include convulsions, loss of consciousness, or feeling disoriented. It's always better to err on the side of caution.

A headache that develops after you've hit your head should be evaluated by your doctor. In some cases bleeding can occur inside your head, a condition called a subdural hematoma or epidural hematoma, and this can be life-threatening. Do not wait to see whether the headache goes away on its own.

If a headache is severe enough to keep you from going about your daily routine, check in with your doctor. This is especially true if you're also feeling dizzy, have blurred vision or other vision changes, fever, or chills.

Check with your doctor if the medication you are using is no longer effective in treating your headaches or if you've developed side effects from the medication.

POINTERS ON PAIN

Always check with the physician when you have a new prescription filled to find out what side effects you are likely to experience.

Diagnosis

Diagnosis of headaches is first based upon your symptoms—what you tell the doctor about when the headache began, what the pain is like, any other symptoms that have come on with the headache, and what you've done to treat it.

Additional diagnostic tools can include an eye exam, blood tests to rule out any medical condition as the cause, discussion of your medical history and any medications you are taking (including vitamins and supplements), discussion of your sleep habits, and if necessary, a neurological examination.

Headaches

Headaches can occur above your eyes or your ears, at the base of your skull, or in back of your upper neck. The pain can be sharp and stabbing or a dull or throbbing ache. You may get a headache rarely, from time to time, or they may be chronic.

Headaches are grouped into three broad categories. Primary and secondary are the first two groupings. The third is sort of a catch-all category and includes cranial neuralgias, pain in the face, and other headaches.

Migraines, cluster, and tension headaches are examples of primary headaches. Secondary headaches are related to a specific medical condition, such as meningitis, a brain tumor, or stroke. The headache you experience when you don't get your morning cup of coffee and are going through caffeine withdrawal is also considered a secondary headache, and so is the headache you can develop with a sinus infection.

Tension Headache

Far and away the most common type of headache is the tension headache. You can blame it on the stress of modern-day living, and you're probably right. They're more common in women than in men, but overall about 90 percent of us will have a tension headache at some point, and some people struggle through them almost on a daily basis.

Tension headaches often feel as if someone were tightening a vise around your head. It's usually a dull ache that affects both sides of your head, although sometimes it can feel as if it's pulsating. It tends to get worse as it progresses.

Because of the stress involved, your shoulders may ache and your head may be overly sensitive to touch. Often when you have such a headache, you keep your shoulders shrugged, causing them to ache as well. This is the kind of headache where it feels as if even the hair on your head is throbbing.

To arrive at a diagnosis of tension headache, the physical exam should produce normal results. You may have some tenderness in your neck or your head, but everything else should come up normal. If other symptoms are evident, then the diagnostic work continues.

SPEAKING OF PAIN

Rebound headaches, or transformed migraines, are a type of tension headache or migraine that occurs when you've overused pain medications over a period of time. The drugs actually cause the headache. Most often these go away or decrease after the medication is stopped.

Tension headaches most often occur in the area of your forehead, your temples, and the base of your skull. They're generally the result of prolonged physical or emotional stress. Some causes of tension headaches include the following:

- Sitting at the computer for extended periods of time, which causes your muscles to tighten up

- Osteoarthritis in your neck or upper spine

- Temporomandibular joint problems

- Prolonged coughing or sneezing

- Excessive physical labor

Depression and anxiety can also bring on tension headaches.

Migraine Headache

You may have heard this referred to as a "sick headache," and it's a good description, as migraines may be accompanied by both nausea and vomiting. Pain is usually on one side of the head and can feel as if it's right behind the eye. It can be dull or throbbing and generally occurs on the same side of the head each time. A hypersensitivity to light, sound, or smell is a classic symptom. Many people pull the shades and keep the lights down low to deal with this symptom. Others go to a quiet, dark room to help deal with the pain.

POINTERS ON PAIN

Distinctive patterns of light, so intense that they can be visually painful, blind spots, blurred or tunnel vision, or pain in an eye may precede a migraine. This change in vision is called an aura.

About 28 million people in the United States get migraines, and this headache comes in right behind tension headaches as the most common kind. In fact, 10 percent of the population suffers with a migraine at some time or other, and they can begin in children younger than eight years old. Most often they affect young and middle-aged adults, primarily women. There also seems to be a genetic predisposition to developing migraine headaches.

Before adolescence, migraines strike both boys and girls in similar numbers, but after the onset of puberty, girls are more affected by them.

There may also be a hormonal component to migraines. Some women get migraines around the time of their monthly period. It's believed that a fluctuation in hormone levels is responsible. Interestingly, during the later stages of pregnancy, women often experience fewer migraines than they did before they became pregnant.

What causes migraines? Researchers are still unsure, although they tend to think now that certain nerve pathways in the brain are responsible. Somehow chemical reactions take place that disturb the normal functioning of these nerves.

If you are susceptible, migraines can be triggered by stress, physical exercise, or changes in eating and sleeping patterns. Other triggers include the following:

- Use of alcohol

- Certain fragrances, such as perfumes or room deodorizers

- Smoking or exposure to second-hand smoke

- Bright light—either sunlight or artificial light

- Loud noise

- Dehydration

- Skipping meals

It's also possible that migraines can result from an allergic reaction to specific foods or chemicals used as preservatives in certain foods. The list is extensive:

- Foods containing nitrates (found in dried and cured meats such as bacon, hot dogs, and salami)

- Foods containing monosodium glutamate (MSG), used as a flavor enhancer—especially in Chinese food

- Foods containing tyramine (found in red wine, aged cheese, chicken livers, figs, and some beans)

- Foods that have been smoked, fermented or pickled, marinated, or processed in any way

Specific foods that can trigger a migraine headache include chocolate, dairy products, baked goods, onions, peanut butter and other nuts, citrus fruits, avocados, and bananas.

Migraines can last from several hours to two or more days, and after the headache has passed, you may find yourself exhausted, have difficulty concentrating, and crave sleep.

Diagnosis is made by explaining your symptoms to the doctor, analyzing your medical history, and undergoing a physical examination. In some cases, your doctor may recommend an EEG, MRI, or CT scan to rule out other causes.

STABS AND JABS

A double whammy! Mixed tension migraine headaches combine the worst features of migraine and tension headaches. These tend to affect women more than men.

Cluster Headache

Men are more affected by cluster headaches than are women. This type of headache comes on each day for a period of several days, weeks, or months. Sometimes they can be seasonal, appearing in the spring, for example. These headaches can begin during childhood but are most common in men between 20 to 40 years of age.

Cluster headaches generally have a predictable pattern, and they can be excruciatingly painful. Symptoms include the following:

- Pain is centered around one eye and limited to one side of the face.
- The affected eye may be watery and inflamed.
- The nostril on the side that's affected may become congested or runny.
- Headaches develop a pattern—developing around the same time each day.

If your cluster headaches begin during the night, the pain will wake you, and lying in bed will seem to make the headache worse. While you're in the cluster pattern you may find you develop a headache once or twice a day, and sometimes more often than that. Cluster headaches typically last from 15 to 45 minutes, although some can last longer.

Several risk factors and triggers have been discovered for cluster headaches. There seems to be a genetic connection, so the tendency to develop cluster headaches may be inherited.

Certain medications or substances that dilate blood vessels can precipitate cluster headaches. One example is nitroglycerin, taken for coronary artery disease. Alcohol is another substance that dilates blood vessels, so it, too, may trigger an attack. If you are in the midst of a cluster sequence, you may find that smoking can trigger an attack.

Anything that disrupts your normal routine can be a trigger for headache in some people. This can include changes in your sleeping schedule or bouts of insomnia. Even changes in the environment may be responsible for generating headaches if you're susceptible to them. These changes can be shifts in barometric pressure, along with the weather changes that accompany these shifts.

POINTERS ON PAIN

If you're traveling and are in the midst of a cluster pattern, know that changes in altitude can trigger an attack.

Just as with tension and migraine headaches, diagnosis is based upon your disclosure of your symptoms. Headaches that occur like clockwork and are accompanied by excruciating pain are classic symptoms of cluster headache. If you're having an attack during the doctor visit, your tearing eye and stuffy or runny nose help confirm the diagnosis.

Occipital Neuralgia

This type of headache gets its name from the occipital nerves, which are located where your spinal column and neck connect and which then travel up to your scalp at the back of your head. Occipital neuralgia is piercing, throbbing, and can feel like electric shocks converging at your upper neck, the back of your head, and behind your ears and eyes. It usually affects just one side of your head at a time. Your forehead may also hurt, along with your scalp. As with a migraine, you may find that light is very painful, and you need a darkened room to rest.

Occipital neuralgia has numerous causes that include the following:

- Accident or a blow to the back of the head

- Compression of the occipital nerve as it leaves the spine (a result of osteoarthritis)

- Tight neck muscles

- Tumors or nodules in the neck

- Inflammation or infection in the neck

- Poor posture (holding your head forward and down for long periods of time

Underlying medical conditions that can cause this type of headache include diabetes, gout, and inflammation of the blood vessels (vasculitis). In some cases, there is no apparent trigger for occipital neuralgia.

Diagnosis is made by an evaluation of your symptoms and a physical examination. A nerve block that provides relief from pain is sometimes used to confirm a diagnosis of occipital neuralgia.

Post-Concussive Headache

Football players get them. So do accident victims. This type of headache generally results from a blow to the head or other trauma that causes a concussion. Symptoms are generally a throbbing headache and neck pain that persist over time, coupled with dizziness and feelings of disorientation. The severity of the headache is not necessarily related to the severity of the accident or trauma that caused it.

SPEAKING OF PAIN

The Centers for Disease Control (CDC) report that each year more than 1.4 million concussions occur in the United States. That's a lot of headaches.

Post-concussive headache is diagnosed by an evaluation of symptoms, physical examination, and medical history that includes details of the trauma sustained prior to the headache's onset. In some cases, imaging tests may be used to detect any bleeding in the brain or other abnormalities responsible for the pain.

Prevention

Preventing headaches is definitely preferable to treating them after they've struck. The first step is learning about your headaches. You can begin by keeping a headache diary to see what your triggers are. (See Chapter 3 for a complete discussion of pain profiles.) After you've identified your triggers, you can take steps to reduce their frequency or impact.

For reducing the frequency of tension headaches, consider wearing a mouthpiece (similar to what's prescribed for treating temporomandibular jaw disorder—see "Temporomandibular Jaw Disorder" later in this chapter) at night. This takes stress away from your jaw so it relaxes instead of tensing up.

You can also help prevent headaches by keeping yourself fit. This means getting enough sleep, exercising regularly, and learning how to manage stress so that it doesn't manage you. You'll find some good suggestions for doing this in Chapter 8.

Preventing post-concussive headache involves taking appropriate safety precautions when playing contact sports (wearing helmets, face protectors, and other protective gear), and buckling up when driving.

Treatment

Sooner is better than later when treating headaches. Tension headaches generally respond well to over-the-counter analgesics. If your tension headaches are difficult to manage, your physician may prescribe an antidepressant medication. These have proven effective in reducing both the frequency and the duration of tension headaches.

For a migraine, drink plenty of water to keep yourself hydrated. Rest in a darkened room, and place a cool cloth or an ice pack at the base of your skull or on the side of the temple that is pulsating. Some people find it beneficial to press the pulsating temple with their own fingers or have a loved one massage that area. Others don't want to be touched by anyone!

Prescription medications are available to reduce the frequency of your attacks. These include seizure or blood pressure medications and certain antidepressants. Although you may not have the primary condition these medications were designed to treat, one happy side effect of them is their ability to work on migraine headaches.

After you've got an active migraine, you may get relief from over-the-counter pain medications, such as aspirin, ibuprofen, or acetaminophen. If these aren't effective, don't increase the dosage beyond recommended levels. Instead, call your physician, as prescription medications are available as well. These come in tablet, injection, or nasal spray form.

Imitrex is one prescription medication that's proven effective in treating migraine as well as cluster headache, for which it's generally given as an injection. Other prescription medications include Migranal (dihydroergotamine), Sandostatin, and Sandostatin LAR (octreotide).

Feverfew is an herb that's been used for many years to prevent or treat migraines. You may find it helps you. You can grow your own or find it at health food stores or pharmacies.

> **STABS AND JABS**
>
> Do you know what's in that pill? Herbs and supplements are not regulated by the FDA. You cannot be sure, therefore, about their quality, safety, or even if they contain what the labels say they do.

Cluster headaches can be difficult to treat without prescription medications. These come in tablet, injection, or nasal spray form. Oxygen is also used to treat cluster headaches and in some cases works to prevent an attack.

For occipital neuralgia, heat, rest, and massage can be helpful. Other treatments include muscle relaxants, anti-inflammatory medications, and local nerve blocks.

When post-concussive headache does not respond to over-the-counter or prescription medications, further evaluation of this condition by your physician or neurologist is indicated.

Headaches are far and away the most common type of head pain, but injuries to the head, infections, and certain medical conditions can also cause pain.

Whiplash

Whiplash is the commonly used term to describe a soft-tissue injury to the neck, usually as the result of an automobile accident. The neck snaps forward and then back quickly. This injury is discussed in Chapter 11.

The headache that results from a whiplash injury is diagnosed with a physical examination and evaluation of symptoms. Occasionally, imaging tests may be suggested, if the headache does not respond to treatment with over-the-counter or nonsteroidal anti-inflammatory drugs (NSAIDs).

Sinus Pain: When "Nothing" Hurts

This type of pain often begins as pressure between your eyes, behind your nose, or in your forehead or cheeks. Sometimes your teeth will hurt. Your sinuses are cavities, and these cavities can become inflamed, infected, and congested. When that happens, the cavities fill with fluid—the mucus that's supposed to drain down through your nasal passages.

You feel this congestion most severely when you lie down. Nothing is draining; instead, it's all backing up, and it gets painful. So in the simplest terms, you can blame a sinus headache on congested sinuses.

Other symptoms of sinus pain include fatigue and fever or chills. Also, this type of headache tends to last longer than other kinds.

Causes of this congestion run the gamut from a head cold or allergies all the way to infection of some type. If the congestion doesn't seem to be showing signs of getting better after a week, you may have developed an infection (sinusitis) in your sinuses, and the headache that goes along with it just doesn't get better either.

Treatment

For minor sinus congestion you can try an over-the-counter oral or nasal decongestant and also use a saline nasal spray. This works by thinning the thick mucus and allowing it to drain more easily. Antihistamines will help if your sinus headache is caused by allergies.

Over-the-counter pain relievers, such as ibuprofen or acetaminophen, can be helpful, but to avoid overdosing, be sure you're not already getting these ingredients in any other over-the-counter medications.

Moisture can help with the symptoms of sinus pain. A mist humidifier can be beneficial, as can a warm steam spa. If you don't have either of these, step into the shower and turn the water on warm. Close the doors and breathe in the warm, humid air.

Afterward, lying down and alternating hot and cold compresses to your face can also reduce the discomfort.

If you're still having congestion after three weeks, the condition can be called chronic sinusitis and prescription medication, such as an antibiotic or antifungal medication, is generally needed to get rid of it.

Surgery

When sinus infections become chronic, and the pain is almost constant, and you are not getting relief with medications, you may want to consider surgery. An *endoscopy* allows the surgeon to remove diseased tissue and restore good drainage to your sinuses with minimally invasive techniques. See Chapter 9 for a complete discussion of this surgical approach.

> **DEFINITION**
>
> **Endoscopy** is a procedure in which a narrow flexible tube equipped with a light and a camera is inserted through a small incision or a natural opening, such as the nostril, to diagnose and allow repair of damaged tissue.

Nerve Pain in the Face

Nerve pain is sharp and stabbing. The medical term for this condition is trigeminal neuralgia, and it's a common type of nerve pain disorder. It tends to affect women over the age of 50 more than men and is usually limited to one side of your face.

The trigeminal nerve, which relays sensory information from your face to your brain, has three branches. Most often the pain involves your cheekbone, nose, upper lip, and top teeth. After that, most other cases involve your lower cheek, lip, and jaw.

> **POINTERS ON PAIN**
>
> Trigeminal neuralgia is commonly known as *tic douloureux,* French for "painful or sad twitching." The nerve twitches, resulting in a facial expression that resembles a grimace.

Finding a cause for trigeminal neuralgia can be difficult. It can develop as the result of an injury, infection, or from blood vessels pressing on the nerve.

The pain is severe, lasting anywhere from a few seconds to several minutes at a time. Because it's erratic, it can disrupt your normal routine, including sleeping and eating. This disruption can lead to malnutrition, dehydration, anxiety, and serious depression.

The lightest touch or vibration can trigger an attack, and when you consider how often your face moves with talking, eating, or drinking, you can see why sufferers would resist anything that causes movement to their faces. This includes hygiene as well (brushing your teeth, washing your face, or shaving). Unfortunately, hospitalization may be required to treat the pain.

Diagnosis is made with a physical and neurological examination, which rules out an underlying medical condition, such as multiple sclerosis, as the cause.

Treatment includes oral medications, especially antiseizure medications that work by suppressing nerve activity. Specific medications to treat trigeminal neuralgia include baclofen (Lioresal), carbamazepine (Tegretol), and phenytoin (Dilantin). If these aren't effective, a nerve block delivered by injection or surgery to decompress or destroy the nerve responsible can be administered.

Pain in Your Mouth

In this section we'll take a look at the three typical areas where pain arises inside your mouth: your teeth, your gums, and the structure that supports them all—your jaw. Sometimes these areas hurt because something is going wrong somewhere else in your body. You can then look at this pain as a symptom or a clue to the real problem.

Toothache

It's not always a simple task to find the source of tooth pain. Most often a cavity, an exposed root, or a cracked or abscessed tooth is responsible, but sometimes the pain isn't coming from the tooth at all. In some cases, tooth pain can be a symptom of a sinus or ear infection. It can also be an early sign of coronary artery disease or even heart attack.

Tooth pain can be a simple ache that's not too difficult to ignore, or it can be sharp and stabbing if a nerve is involved. Diagnosis and treatment takes place at the dentist's office.

Over-the-counter pain relievers can help until you can schedule an appointment with the dentist, but tooth pain is definitely not a "do-it-yourself" type of repair.

Gum Disease

By the time your gums start to hurt, a great deal of damage has already taken place. Over-the-counter pain relievers can help with the pain, but unless you get to the root of the problem, the pain will persist. Make an appointment with your dentist to treat this condition, save your teeth, and relieve your pain.

Temporomandibular Jaw Disorder

Do you grind your teeth when you sleep? You may not be aware of it, except for a sore jaw upon waking. Often tooth-grinding is a result of stress or tension. Your dentist can prescribe a mouthpiece for you to wear when you go to bed. This mouthpiece cushions the space between your upper and lower teeth and keeps them from grinding together.

Injury to the temporomandibular joint (the joint that works as a hinge linking your upper and lower jaw), such as getting hit in the face or being in a car accident, can result in pain to this area. Infection or muscle spasms here can also be the reason for pain.

Over-the-counter anti-inflammatory medications, such as ibuprofen or naproxen, can relieve the pain. If they aren't effective, prescription medications are available from your doctor. Surgery to remove impacted teeth may also provide relief.

The Least You Need to Know

- Headaches that come on suddenly or that are intense require immediate medical attention.
- Most headaches respond to over-the-counter pain relievers. Prescription medications are available if something stronger is necessary.
- Infection in your sinuses can cause headaches. Treating the infection should solve the problem.
- If your gums are painful, see your dentist at once to avoid tooth loss.
- Teeth-grinding and jaw clenching can lead to headache. Your dentist has the answer to your pain.

Neck Pain and Back Pain

In This Chapter

- Understanding why your back or neck hurts
- Changing habits
- Exercise essentials
- The range of treatment options

Injury to any part of the spine can be serious and in some cases life-threatening. Injury can involve damage to your ligaments, muscles, and nerves as well as to the bones in your spine. Sometimes pain in this area is the result of strains and over-worked muscles, but it can also be a symptom of an underlying medical condition. In this chapter, we'll take a look at that pain in your neck, along with your upper back, and give you suggestions for treating it as well as preventing future problems.

When to See the Doctor

You don't want to run to the doctor with every little ache and pain, of course, but sometimes "toughing it out" is not the best course of action. When your pain is accompanied by certain other problems, you need to see the doctor. Call your physician if you are experiencing any of the following:

- Chills or fever
- Pain when you cough
- Weakness in your arms or legs
- Weight loss that you can't account for

- Loss of control of bladder or bowel function

- Inability to go to the bathroom

Common sense needs to be your guide. If you can't function because the pain is so severe or if it's not improving over the course of a few weeks, then it just makes sense to get professional advice.

SPEAKING OF PAIN

Low back pain comes in second only to headache as the most common neurological ailment. According to the National Institute of Neurological Disorders and Stroke, U.S. sufferers from low back pain spend a whopping $50 billion a year treating this condition. Approximately 85 percent of all Americans will experience low back pain during the course of their lifetimes, so you are not alone.

Diagnosis

If you don't recall injuring your back or neck, diagnosis becomes a matter of ruling out other conditions that may be responsible for your pain. The first two steps in this process are a physical examination of you and an examination of your medical history.

Your doctor will ask questions about your back pain—when it started, what you were doing when it started, how severe it is, and whether it is constant or comes and goes. Your pain diary (see Chapter 3 for information on keeping a pain diary) will help you be complete and accurate in answering these questions.

She'll want to know whether the pain is interfering with your ability to get around and whether you've had to cut back on your activities.

If your doctor suspects that an underlying medical condition is causing your pain or feels that waiting isn't likely to result in any improvement, she may recommend blood tests and imaging tests.

Blood tests are used to rule out or discover the presence of certain diseases as the source of your neck or back pain. They will check markers of infections or arthritis such as CRP and rheumatoid factor. Other blood tests to check vitamin D levels, look at your thyroid function, and report your blood sugar reading (to check for diabetes) may also be done.

Blood tests by themselves may not give the whole picture, so your doctor may need imaging tests, such as x-rays, a CT scan, or an MRI, to make the diagnosis (see Chapter 4 for a detailed explanation of blood tests and imaging tests).

Sources of Neck and Back Pain

The big contributors here are accidents and other injuries that harm the muscles, ligaments, tendons, and bones of your spinal column. Most often, patients report the most mundane activity such as twisting or bending over to pick up something caused their neck or low back pain. Certain medical conditions can also cause your neck and back to hurt.

Medical Conditions

Arthritis, poor posture, and radiculopathies (pinched nerves) are the most common medical conditions responsible for neck and back pain. Diabetes, thyroid disease, and vitamin deficiencies are less common causes, while cancer and infection may also cause such pain problems.

Determining which, if any, of these are the culprits requires blood work. Your doctor will most likely request a CBC panel to rule out these possible causes or confirm that one (or more) of them is responsible.

Injury

In addition to sprains and strains, pulled muscles, and torn ligaments, fractures of the spine are a common source of back pain. Many times these are *compression fractures*. Compression fractures of the spine often result from a fall or other accident that jars the spine.

DEFINITION

A **compression fracture** occurs when the vertebrae of the spine are first subjected to severe jarring and then come crashing together. If the force of the impact is hard enough, the bones break.

These compression fractures set the stage for osteoarthritis to develop. The resulting pain can be severe. Older adults may want to get evaluated for osteoporosis if they do suffer a compression fracture.

Aging and the Pull of Gravity

Men and women between the ages of 30 to 50 are the most likely to experience low back pain, and often it's the result of a sedentary lifestyle or an unequal mix of inactivity during the week and excessive activity over the weekend.

As your spine ages, it needs a little tender loving care. The bone can lose density and strength, the muscles supporting your spine lose their youthful elasticity, and even the shock-absorber discs between the vertebrae undergo changes. They lose their ability to spring back quickly and can also lose fluid necessary to keep them supple. Even normal activities can tax the limits of the aging spine.

Narrowing of the Spine

The medical term for narrowing of the spine is spinal stenosis, and it's most often found in people over the age of 50. If you have arthritis of the spine, bone spurs can grow. These bone spurs, along with thickened ligaments (which can occur with arthritis or normal aging), can take up room in the canal, making it smaller. Spinal stenosis can also develop if you have a herniated disc. This condition isn't an easy one to diagnose without imaging tests such as CT scans or MRI.

Slipped Vertebra

Ligaments that hold your spine in place can lose their elasticity and strength, and when this happens, the vertebrae in your spine can shift position. Other causes of this process can be fractures and abnormal curvatures of the spine.

Sometimes, people are born with these slipped vertebrae but don't have symptoms until they are much older. These vertebrae can move so much that they press on the nerves in the spine, creating pain down the buttocks or legs. This condition is called spondylolisthesis. Imaging tests, such as x-rays, are needed to confirm this diagnosis.

Disc Problems

Strong as the discs in your back are, sometimes they develop tears in the outer portion. These tears can sometimes cause pain that can range from mild to severe. Sometimes the pain lasts for a short time, but other times it can become chronic. X-rays and imaging tests are needed to see if you have a tear in your disc.

Sciatica

Sciatica is a term familiar to most people, and it can be an extremely painful condition. Most people use this term to describe a pinched nerve anywhere in the back, but specifically, sciatica refers to one nerve called the sciatic nerve. This nerve runs in the back of the thigh and leg. You may experience pain in your buttock and leg, along with numbness and tingling in the thigh, leg, and foot. Sometimes there can be some weakness in the foot or leg.

Generally, your physical examination and medical history can help your doctor arrive at this diagnosis, although imaging tests may be needed to confirm the diagnosis.

Curvature of the Spine

Curvature of the spine occurs as a developmental problem, rather than as a result of an injury. Your spine isn't a straight-up-and-down structure, but rather has three curves to it.

Sometimes the curves in the spinal column curve more than they should. This condition is called scoliosis, and when it puts pressure on certain nerves, it can cause low back pain and sometimes leg symptoms, such as pain, tingling, or numbness. Children and teenagers can develop scoliosis. Scoliosis screening can detect this condition early on so that corrective measures can be taken. Scoliosis is easily detected on x-rays.

Irritation of the Joints in the Neck and Thorax

Your neck has a range of motion that allows you to move it from side to side, as well as forward. It's not designed to move backward—at least not very much. The good part is that your neck moves easily. The bad part is that your neck moves easily. If your neck is forced beyond its normal, intended range of motion, the muscles and ligaments and tendons in this area are strained.

The most common causes of this kind of injury are a sudden blow, a fall, or an automobile accident. You've undoubtedly heard this type of injury referred to as whiplash, although your doctor may call it a cervical sprain or strain. Sometimes it's also called a hyperextension injury. Regardless of the term used, it's painful. Generally, a physical examination and medical history can provide an accurate diagnosis, although imaging tests may be necessary to determine the extent of the damage.

"Hunchback"

This condition, in which the upper back develops an abnormal rounding, is also known as "dowager's hump." The medical term is kyphosis. Sometimes the rounding isn't apparent to the naked eye, but other times it's quite noticeable. Kyphosis may be diagnosed when the rounding of the upper back is mild or extreme. This is measured in degrees. It's diagnosed with imaging tests, which can include x-rays.

Kyphosis can have many causes and can occur anywhere from infancy to old age. It can be a developmental problem, can result from an injury to the thoracic spine (the part of your spine below your neck), or can be a result of osteoarthritis. It is often caused due to micro-compression of the vertebral body as we age. This does not mean that all of us will eventually get it.

The Strategy of Prevention

An ounce of prevention is worth a pound of medicine. Prevention is also cheaper than surgery, and if you can head off neck and back pain by making some simple (and mostly free) lifestyle changes, you'll be doing yourself and your checkbook a big favor. Most preventive measures center around unlearning some bad habits and learning some good ones.

Improving Your Posture

Poor posture can be a big cause of mechanical back pain. It's easy to fall into bad habits and difficult to break them. Change isn't easy, and changing the way you sit, stand, work, and perform household tasks takes commitment and perseverance.

It's no coincidence that more time spent on the computer translates into more neck, shoulder, and back pain. The cause of upper back and neck pain can be linked to posture. First, though, you need to learn what changes you can make and how to make them.

POINTERS ON PAIN

Your mother's constant reminders to "Stand up straight!" and "Sit up straight!" were right on the money. Slumping and slouching are hard on your back and neck and over time can be the source of ongoing pain.

Keeping the same position for an extended period of time is hard on your back. It can cause muscle strain and fatigue, and with that fatigue comes an increased risk of injury.

At first, correct postures may be uncomfortable. The reason is that the muscles and ligaments have stretched in some places (the incorrect ones) and shortened and tightened in other places (the correct ones). Bringing them back to their normal positions puts tension and some strain on them, which can cause you some discomfort until things are back to where they belong. In the meantime, you're going to need to be on constant alert to maintain proper postures. It won't help much if you straighten up only now and then.

You've got to develop a sense of body awareness and learn to be mindful of your postures. In the beginning, maintaining this awareness can be very difficult, but eventually you won't even notice.

Practice Correct Posture

Practice is important to maintaining correct posture. Place a reminder note by your computer to sit up straight, tuck your chin down, pull your shoulders back, relax your elbows, and tighten your abdominal muscles. Don't forget to take frequent stretching breaks—one every 30 to 45 minutes would be ideal.

Check your posture in a full-length mirror. First, stand the way you normally do and critique yourself. It is really important to look at yourself from the side as well. This helps you see the alignment of your head, chin, and shoulders. Are your shoulders hunched over or turned in too much? Does gravity seem to be dragging you down so that your rib cage is settling in over your abdomen? Does your chin extend forward, and does your bottom pull back too much?

If you notice any of these posture faults, the remedy is to straighten your shoulders. Raise them and slightly rotate them backwards until your rib cage lifts and you can take a deep, cleansing breath of air. As your rib cage expands and lifts, your spine falls into a more normal alignment. Your goal is to make this posture your normal posture. Practice standing tall and erect and see how much better you feel. Your feet should be slightly spread apart, in line with your shoulders.

Shoulder and back posture supports are available at medical supply stores and also online. These supports are worn under your clothing and help correct posture problems by gently moving your muscles into the correct position. But be careful—not all supports are best for all body types and postures. Check with your physician or physical therapist to be sure you're not doing more harm than good!

> **SPEAKING OF PAIN**
>
> It takes about three weeks to change a habit, and poor posture is a habit. During this time your brain has to unlearn a bad habit and replace it with a new one. You can't rush the process. Be patient and practice, and you'll be successful.

Raise your head and tuck in your chin! Slumping posture puts your eyes at floor level, so hold your head up and let your eyes connect to a point straight ahead. If your chin is on a line parallel with the floor, you're doing this posture correctly.

To test your accuracy, try to balance a hardcover book on top of your head. Nothing too heavy, though, and be sure it's resting on the flat part of your skull top. If the book slides forward, raise your chin a bit and try again until you're successful at keeping it there. That's the position you're going to work at perfecting.

Change Positions Frequently

Even after you've learned to sit and stand with good posture, it's important to change positions frequently during the day.

If you've been sitting, stand and stretch. If you've been standing, sit down. These variations in position become even more important if you have a congenital back deformity, such as scoliosis.

Changing positions takes the pressure off specific muscles and ligaments and gives them the necessary time to recuperate. This "down time" helps them perform more efficiently, keeps you from getting fatigued, and helps prevent pain.

Improving Your Posture While Driving

Driving to and from work, to the store, or on vacation, Americans spend hours behind the wheel. Those hours can be stressful on your back and cause you pain, if your posture isn't correct. The problem centers around the position of the driver's seat and your position in it.

Once again, sitting up straight is key. If you hunch your shoulders forward to grasp the wheel or recline your seat so that your arms must stretch to reach the wheel, you're straining your back and neck muscles. Also, if you've pushed your seat too far forward you could hurt your back, hips, and knees.

You should be able to place your hands comfortably in the 10 and 2 o'clock positions on the steering wheel, with elbows slightly bent. Your knees should also be bent slightly as you work the floor pedals. If your legs are stretched to the max, you're putting strain on your lower back.

STABS AND JABS

Whiplash is an extremely painful injury, and not using your headrest properly can make it even more so. The back of your head should rest against the cushioned part of the headrest.

Improving Your Posture at the Office

Ergonomically designed office chairs can take some of the pressure off your entire back, as you work at the computer or at your desk. They are a good idea for the home office as well, since their curves correspond to the natural curvature of the spine. After you've got such a chair—use it correctly! It won't do you much good if you perch on the edge of the seat and don't take maximum advantage of the chair's design.

If your neck is bothering you and you can't pinpoint the reason for your pain, it might be your telephone that's causing the problem. More accurately, the way you're holding the phone might be the problem. Devices that allow you to position the phone between your neck and your shoulder, so your hands remain free, put strain on your neck and are a common source of neck pain. The solution? Either hold the phone with your hand or use a hands-free device so you can simply push a button and talk without involving your neck and shoulder.

Carrying and Lifting Correctly

Carrying a shoulder bag by having the weight suspended from just one shoulder throws your spine out of alignment and can cause muscle strain and pain. If you carry a shoulder bag, place the strap so it falls diagonally across your chest. This distributes the bag's weight more evenly across your body. An added benefit to this arrangement is security. Holding the bag closer to your body is a deterrent to purse snatchers.

When you carry heavy items, use your forearms rather than your hands to support the bulk of the weight. The more body surface you bring to a task, the more evenly the weight is distributed and the less strain you put on specific muscles. When you just use your hand, the weight is pulling your arm down, and this strain can travel all the way to your neck and upper back.

It's surprising, but even lifting relatively light items can throw your back out of whack and cause serious pain. Don't combine twisting and lifting. This is a typical cause of severe back pain. Instead, position yourself so you can lift the item first and then move your body in the necessary orientation to complete the maneuver.

When you lift, lift with your knees, not your back. Make sure you don't lift without squatting first. Use your legs and thighs to help with the weight and remember to keep the load close to your body. The closer the load, the less the strain. Get in the habit now, before you have problems, and you may never have to feel that excruciating stab of pain that's letting you know you lifted the wrong way.

If your job requires you to lift, be sure to wear the back support that you're issued. OSHA has provided specific safety measures that companies must follow to ensure that their employees reduce the risk of injuring themselves from lifting. When you must lift something, the back or hernia brace protects the muscles and ligaments in your lower back.

POINTERS ON PAIN

For women: High-heeled shoes throw your back out of alignment and create all kinds of havoc with your spine. Switch to low heels that keep your spine in the proper alignment, and you'll save your back.

One last helpful hint for moving heavy objects so that you put the least amount of strain on your back muscles and ligaments: push rather than pull. Forward motion is much easier on your body than backward motion because pulling forces your spine backward—making it vulnerable to injury.

Sleeping Positions

Your spine has natural curves. A mattress is flat. Right away you can see the possibility for compatibility issues. Sleeping on your back puts strain on your spine—you're pulling it out of alignment. This is a common reason for morning back pain.

If you like to sleep on your back, place a pillow under your knees to relieve the strain. Make sure your pillow doesn't have a high loft, as this puts strain on your upper back and neck. If you're a side sleeper, place a pillow between your knees to keep your spine aligned properly.

Mattresses that are too soft or that sag are very hard on your back. Invest in a good-quality mattress and choose one that's firmer as opposed to softer. Even good mattresses have a natural life span and will need to be replaced with a new one every few years.

> **POINTERS ON PAIN**
>
> Foam supports for your neck and back can be found at most bed and bath stores. Neck supports, called cervical supports, fit inside your pillowcase. Back supports, called lumbar supports, go around your waist and support the lower curve as you sleep.

Watch Your Weight

Being overweight can greatly increase your risk of developing all types of pain, and especially low back pain. The reasons aren't difficult to figure out.

Most overweight people aren't physically active, and they don't eat a healthy, nutritious diet. This means that muscle tone is often poor, and there's not a great deal of flexibility as a result.

If your spine has to spend most of its time and strength supporting your excess weight, you're putting more demands on it than it was designed to take. Some experts think that each extra pound on your belly translates into three extra pounds your back must support.

Maintaining a proper weight is one of the most important good deeds you can do to help your spine do its job effectively. You'll also reduce your risk of developing osteoarthritis in your spine. (See Chapter 21 for a more detailed explanation or check out *The Complete Idiot's Guide to Arthritis*.)

Exercise

You know that exercise is good for you. If you're a regular exerciser, keep it up! If you're not, and if the thought of lacing up your walking shoes or heading to the treadmill or the swimming pool doesn't appeal, consider the following benefits.

- Regular exercise can increase bone strength, muscle flexibility, and endurance.

- Exercise helps you manage your weight, and keeping at an optimal weight decreases stress on your lower back.

- Exercise can decrease your chance of developing osteoporosis.

- Exercise can help alleviate the symptoms of arthritis, a major cause of pain in your spinal vertebrae.

- Exercise can elevate your mood and give you energy to perform your daily tasks with less stress.

Exercise is beneficial for both prevention and treatment of back pain. The exercises recommended for prevention and treatment, however, are different—as is the level of intensity and the number of repetitions.

Your physical therapist (see "Physical Therapy" later in this chapter) can work with you to develop an exercise program specifically tailored to your needs.

POINTERS ON PAIN

Always consult with your physician before beginning any exercise program. This is essential if you're experiencing ongoing back pain, as the incorrect exercises can cause more harm than help.

The muscles that support your back are located in your back, your abdomen, and your buttocks, and keeping these muscles strong and flexible is your first line of defense against back pain. Stretching exercises are good warm-ups but are even better for cool-downs. Walking and swimming are excellent choices for increasing blood flow and stamina and are generally considered safe for nearly everyone.

As with any new venture, begin slowly. Don't overdo at the beginning. Gradually increase the amount of time and level of intensity of your exercise program. Depending on the diagnosis of your back pain, several different types of exercises will be beneficial. Your physical therapist will be the best person to help you find the exercises that will help you the most.

Walking is the best form of exercise. Swift-paced walking helps prevent back aches and other pain problems all over the body. To achieve a cardiovascular exercise with walking, a heart rate monitor is recommended. The heart rate monitor can help you understand what pace you need to walk so that you can get a good workout. To determine your target heart rate, subtract your current age from 220. Then multiply the result by .5 to get the correct number. Do the same calculation (220 – age) × 0.7 and try not to go over this as the maximum heart rate, unless you are already extremely fit.

You should do your exercises for 20 to 30 minutes four times per week, but not as a weekend warrior. If you are not used to such vigorous activity, start slowly. Also, before embarking on any cardiovascular-intensive exercises, check with your primary care physician.

> **SPEAKING OF PAIN**
>
> According to the National Institutes of Health, the first incidence of low back pain is likely to strike people between the ages of 30 and 50.

Exercises that strengthen your abdominal muscles can help prevent back pain. Strong abdominal muscles form a natural support for your lower back. Besides strengthening the rectus abdominis muscles, which we do when we do sit-ups, the transverse abdominis muscle is one to pay close attention to as well. A common way to strengthen the abdomen is to do exercises called pelvic tilts. These exercises can be done while standing, lying down, or sitting.

Treatment for Neck and Back Pain

Sometimes prevention just isn't enough to avoid neck or back pain. If you've suffered an injury, you may need medication, physical therapy, complementary and alternative therapies, or sometimes surgery to feel better. If your pain has been found to be the result of an infection or a symptom of an underlying medical condition, it's time to explore your treatment options.

After you've gone through the testing process, you're ready to discuss a treatment protocol with your physician. The good news is that surgery is almost never the first choice. The better news is that you have many options to consider. The ultimate goal is to get you back into your daily routine and prevent future problems with your back or your neck.

Besides medication to deal with the pain, your physician may also recommend physical therapy to help you achieve greater functionality.

If your back or neck pain is mechanical in origin, meaning that it's the result of injury, stress, or strain, as opposed to being a symptom of an underlying medical condition, you can do a great deal to help yourself heal, relieve your pain, and prevent future problems.

Medications

A variety of prescription and over-the-counter medications are available to treat both acute and chronic neck and back pain. (See Chapter 5 for a complete discussion of these medications.)

The most commonly prescribed medications include nonsteroidal anti-inflammatory drugs (NSAIDs) and acetaminophen. Some NSAIDs include aspirin, ibuprofen, and naprosyn. In addition to providing pain relief, these medications help relieve inflammation, swelling, and general stiffness. Again, NSAIDs can cause severe abdominal and reflux problems along with ulcers, even when taken for a short course. Ask your physician if you should take medications to help your gastrointestinal system remain protected while you're on any NSAID.

Severe, acute pain that doesn't respond to NSAIDs or acetaminophen may be treated with other medications such as pain killers and muscle relaxants. These medications are usually recommended in situations where your daily life is suffering to the point that you can't do the things in your home or work that are required of you. These medications are also used best when used temporarily.

Topical preparations, such as lotions, sprays, or creams, can be applied to the skin. These help relieve pain by creating counter-sensations of warmth or of cold and work by stimulating nerve endings in the skin.

Physical Therapy

If your pain is the result of an injury or a spinal deformity, such as scoliosis, your physician may recommend that you work with a physical therapist to help strengthen your back muscles.

Physical therapy has two purposes: to help you heal and to teach you strategies that will enable you to avoid re-injuring your back. But physical therapy is only as good as you are compliant. This means you have to take what you learn in therapy and practice it on your own.

At your first session, you'll meet your therapist and spend some time discussing the nature of your injury or medical condition and define your goals for physical therapy—regaining flexibility, improving your posture, strengthening and stretching your back muscles, and learning how to avoid future injury.

Your physical therapist will most likely conduct some tests to determine what movements you can perform without pain and which ones cause you pain. This will help in creating your personalized therapy program.

POINTERS ON PAIN

It's important to remember that a certain amount of discomfort doesn't always mean that an exercise is harmful to you. Sometimes it means that the exercise is getting to the heart of the problem. Tell your therapist when it hurts and how much.

You'll also develop a schedule for your appointments and receive instruction on what to do at home to continue your therapy.

Complementary and Alternative Therapies

Stress and tension can make back pain more severe. Learning how to manage stress and reduce tension can help relieve your pain as well as prevent pain. Often, an integrated approach to managing neck and back pain is the most productive, and you may find acupuncture, massage, or chiropractic treatment helpful additions to your therapy.

Local hospitals, community centers, YMCAs, or senior centers often sponsor classes in stress management and weight management, and offer a variety of educational and recreational opportunities, including tai chi, dance, or other classes that are either free or offered at nominal cost.

Surgery

No one looks forward to surgery, but some back conditions may benefit from it. Generally, surgery is not indicated for back pain, unless the pain is caused by a fracture, a tumor, or an infection. If you've experienced weakness or bowel and bladder problems, surgery may help. Surgery may be recommended in the following situations.

- If you have a ruptured (herniated or slipped) disc, surgery to remove that disc may be indicated.

- If your spine has become unstable as the result of an injury to the spinal vertebrae or because of a spinal tumor, or if you have a congenital spinal defect, such as scoliosis, your surgeon may recommend spinal fusion to stabilize your spine.

- If you have developed spinal stenosis as a result of the aging process, relieving pressure on the spinal nerves by removing some bone or thickened ligaments inside the spinal column and giving the nerves inside more space may be recommended to help you walk more.

You'll find a complete discussion of surgeries in Chapter 9.

The Least You Need to Know

- Neck and back pain can result from injury or be a sign of an underlying medical condition or a developmental problem.
- Lifestyle changes, medication, and physical therapy can often help relieve back and neck pain.
- Developing good posture is both your best pain relief tactic and your best preventive measure against back and neck pain.
- Maintaining a proper weight is one of the best means of preventing low back pain.
- Alternative therapies such as massage, acupuncture, and chiropractic can be helpful additions to your pain treatment protocol.

Chest Pain

Chapter 12

In This Chapter

- Is your heart to blame?
- Fear and pain
- Problems with arteries
- Rib injuries

Chest pain can be an unnerving experience. Your first thought may be that you're having a heart attack, but the reality is that a heart attack is just one possibility. Sometimes the pain can be due to an injury, infection, your state of mind, and even your gender! Chest pain is nothing to fool around with, and it's definitely not a good idea to be your own physician here. In this chapter, we'll cover the basics of how you can get relief when your chest hurts.

When to See the Doctor

Pain or pressure in your chest—what's been described as "an elephant sitting on your chest"—requires immediate medical attention. If you are experiencing shortness of breath, nausea, dizziness, or if the pain is going to your jaw or down your arm or to your neck, you may be having a heart attack.

Sometimes these symptoms come on gradually. You may have some or all of them, and they may come and go. Does this mean that everyone experiencing such symptoms is having a heart attack? No, but only a physician can determine what the source of the problem is. In any case, a "wait and see" attitude can be fatal. Dial 911 for help.

Diagnosis

Whether you've ended up in the emergency room with acute symptoms or are in your doctor's office with less severe symptoms, the medical workup to figure out what is going on is essentially the same.

Your symptoms can give the first clue as to the source of your pain. Then a physical examination can help establish a diagnosis. During the physical examination, your physician will listen carefully to your lungs and heart in addition to checking your abdomen for tenderness and checking for any signs of bulging blood vessels.

POINTERS ON PAIN

In dealing with chest pain, time is of the essence, and treatment may begin before the diagnosis procedure is complete.

In addition to the usual pulse and blood pressure check, you'll have blood work done to check the levels of certain enzymes in your bloodstream and have the oxygen level (oxygen saturation) in your blood measured. Other diagnostic imaging tests may also be ordered.

Electrocardiogram (ECG or EKG)

This test measures the electrical activity of your heart. The physician or technician will attach electrodes to your skin. These electrodes then transmit your heart's electrical impulses to the machine, which shows them as a series of waves on the monitor. This report allows your doctor to determine if your heart is operating normally or if damage has occurred. It can also tell whether any arrhythmia or abnormal beating of the heart is currently occurring.

Angiogram (Coronary Catheterization)

This test measures how well the arteries in your heart are functioning and is useful for locating the point or points of any blockage. A catheter with a tiny camera attached is inserted into an artery, usually the artery in your groin, and from there it's moved up through that artery to your heart. A contrast material is then delivered via the catheter to the arteries in your heart, and the pattern of dye dispersal is monitored on a computer screen.

Other tests include the following:

- Endoscopy
- X-rays
- Nuclear medicine scan
- Electron Beam Computerized Tomography (EBCT) to check for calcium in your arteries
- Echocardiogram

All of these tests help doctors look for abnormalities in the arteries or other structures of your heart.

Stress Test

This can be part of your physical examination to check on your heart health, but it's also used to detect abnormalities in your heart's functioning if you're experiencing chest pain.

As the name implies, this test puts your heart under stress to determine whether it's operating normally when extra demands are put upon it. A treadmill or a stationary bicycle is often used for a stress test.

Electrodes are attached to your skin and are hooked up to the electrocardiogram (ECG). As you exercise, the readings are displayed on a computer monitor.

Not all patients can tolerate the exercise part of the stress test. The physician will make that determination. For those who can't do the exercise, a chemical stress test can be given that stresses the heart without exercise.

Sources of Chest Pain

Your chest area includes the heart and vessels that comprise the cardiovascular system (also known as your circulatory system), the lungs and tissue that make up your respiratory system, and even the portion involved with the digestive system. Therefore, "chest pain" can stem from problems in any of these systems.

In addition to these systems are bones, muscles, tendons, ligaments, and joints. Trauma or illness to any of these parts can cause chest pain. Finding the source of this pain is often a matter of ruling out some possibilities and then closing in on a correct diagnosis. This can take some time.

Heart Attack

The medical term for a heart attack is myocardial infarction. The heart is a muscle, and it needs oxygen to live. In most cases a heart attack occurs as a result of coronary artery disease (CAD) in which deposits of cholesterol, called plaque, build up over time along the walls of the coronary arteries, which are responsible for delivering blood and nutrients to the heart.

If one of these plaques ruptures, it creates a blood clot that can block the artery. Without this blood supply, the part of the heart muscle served by the vessel dies or gets damaged. This is one cause of a heart attack.

STABS AND JABS

Without medical treatment, the heart's electrical impulses may become erratic after a heart attack, a potentially life-threatening condition.

Symptoms of a heart attack may include the following:

- Chest pain—any kind
- Crushing sensation in the chest
- Feelings of intense pressure in the chest
- Pain that radiates into the jaw or arms
- Nausea
- Dizziness
- Shortness of breath
- Heartburn

In women, symptoms of a heart attack may be different from the classic symptoms experienced by men. Pain is still the most common symptom, but fatigue, sweating, or lightheadedness may also be indicators, along with upper back pain or abdominal pain. It should be noted that these atypical symptoms can also be experienced by men who are having a cardiac event.

Risk factors for a heart attack include having high blood pressure and high cholesterol (coronary artery disease), along with a history of smoking or diabetes. In addition, genetics may play a role, as coronary artery disease tends to run in families.

Knowing your risk factors can help you take preventive steps to reduce your chances of heart attack. These steps include quitting smoking, exercising regularly, maintaining a proper weight, and managing your diabetes. Blood pressure and cholesterol-lowering medications may be necessary to get these numbers back within normal limits.

Angina

With angina, the arteries delivering blood to the heart can narrow. This reduced capacity causes a feeling of tightness, pressure, or chest pain. These symptoms are usually associated with physical activity or emotional stress. The symptoms of angina are similar to those of a heart attack. Angina in itself is not a disease but rather it is a symptom of CAD.

SPEAKING OF PAIN

The term given to plaque buildup in your arteries that causes them to narrow is atherosclerosis.

Diagnostic procedures, risk factors, and prevention strategies for angina are the same as for heart attack. Many treatment options are also the same. Medications that dilate blood vessels, blood thinners, and beta blockers to regulate the heartbeat may also be prescribed.

The three basic types of angina are as follows:

- **Stable angina.** This is the most common form and is triggered generally by physical activity or when the heart is working harder than normal. It often has a consistent pattern. If your physician tells you that you have this form of angina, you can often predict what will trigger symptoms for you. Symptoms improve when the trigger is removed or by taking angina medications.

- **Unstable angina.** Pain can be severe with unstable angina. This is a medical emergency. Unstable angina is not predictable and does not follow a predictable pattern. It can occur with or without any physical activity and may not be relieved by rest or medications. This set of conditions may predict an oncoming cardiac event (heart attack) and requires immediate medical attention.

- **Variant angina.** This is the rarest type. It often occurs while at rest. This type of angina is usually controlled with medications.

It's important to understand what circumstances trigger your angina so that you can develop a plan to deal with them. Managing stress and learning what level of physical activity you can engage in are essential components of stress management for angina.

SPEAKING OF PAIN

Angina affects almost seven million people in the United States. It affects men and women in equal proportions.

Inflammation of the Sac Surrounding the Heart

Pericarditis is the medical term for the inflammation of the sac that surrounds your heart. When this sac becomes inflamed, the pain tends to occur in the center of your chest. The pain can be sharp and severe and may be accompanied by fever and a sense of malaise. The pain is caused by the inflamed sac rubbing against the heart's surface. It tends to get worse when you lie down and feels better when you bend forward.

Sometimes the cause of pericarditis can't be determined, and in this case it's said to be idiopathic. Other times, it can be traced to a prior viral illness or be a complication of rheumatoid arthritis, *systemic lupus erythematosus* (*SLE*), certain forms of cancer, or kidney disease. Pericarditis can also result from trauma, such as a car accident in which your chest hits the steering wheel.

DEFINITION

Systemic lupus erythematosus (SLE), commonly called *lupus,* is a chronic inflammatory disease that can affect the joints as well as internal organs, including the kidneys, heart, and lungs.

Diagnosis can be made based upon symptoms, physical examination, and often with diagnostic testing. In some cases, the physician may actually be able to use a stethoscope to hear the sounds of rubbing made by the sac against the heart. But that's not always the case. Diagnostic imaging tests, such as an ECG or a CT scan, are used to confirm the diagnosis.

Nonsteroidal anti-inflammatory drugs (NSAIDs), such as naproxen or ibuprofen, may be prescribed to reduce the inflammation and relieve the pain. In addition, treating the underlying medical condition, if there is one, may help relieve the symptoms.

Pain from a Damaged Aortic Artery

This condition is called an aortic dissection, and it means that the aortic artery actually separates. In an aortic dissection, the inner layers of the aortic artery (the one that leads from your heart) come apart, and blood is forced between them. The pain is severe and comes on suddenly. Aortic dissection is an emergency situation and requires immediate medical assistance.

A variety of conditions can lead to aortic dissection, including high blood pressure, pregnancy, and kidney disease. Cocaine use has also been implicated in aortic dissection.

POINTERS ON PAIN

People with Ehlers-Danlos or Marfan syndrome are at increased risk for aortic dissection.

Heartburn

Heartburn and its companion, acid indigestion, account for a considerable amount of common chest pain. Its major symptom is a burning sensation in the middle of your chest, and the burning is often accompanied with acid-tasting belching.

What distinguishes heartburn from a more immediately serious condition, such as a heart attack, is its timing. It generally develops shortly after you've eaten a meal high in fat. You may feel pain when you swallow and when you lean forward or lie down.

Treatment with an over-the-counter or prescription antacid or stomach acid blocker is usually effective in relieving the pain of heartburn. Frequent heartburn, defined as one or more occurrences a week, however, needs to be evaluated by your physician. You may be referred to a *gastroenterologist* for treatment.

DEFINITION

A **gastroenterologist** is a physician who specializes in diagnosing and treating disorders of the gastrointestinal tract. This tract includes the esophagus, stomach, small and large intestines, pancreas, liver, and gallbladder.

Your doctor may recommend you make some changes in your diet. If heartburn becomes chronic, there is a risk of scarring and subsequent narrowing of the esophagus. Surgery may be necessary to prevent this.

Panic Attack and Panic Symptoms

The mind-body connection is powerful. If you suffer from panic attacks, you are well aware of the physical symptoms they can cause. Panic attacks are considered a true medical condition, defined as a sudden intense situation causing great fear. It may feel as if you are having a heart attack. You may even be afraid you are dying. Along with the intense panic, you may experience chest pain, shortness of breath, sweating, dry mouth, and other symptoms associated with a heart attack.

Treatment includes learning relaxation techniques and having counseling to discover the cause of the panic attacks and then developing strategies for dealing with the situations that bring them on. Antidepressant medications may also be prescribed.

SPEAKING OF PAIN

Ouch! Not all chest pain originates in your chest. Gallbladder and pancreas diseases can cause what is known as referred chest pain.

Inflammation of the Chest Cavity Membrane

When the membrane lining your chest cavity becomes inflamed, a condition known as pleurisy, you may feel sharp pain that gets worse when you take a breath or when you cough. Usually there's an underlying medical condition that's responsible. These can include the following:

- Viral infection

- Pneumonia

- Tuberculosis

- Cancer

- Kidney failure

- Autoimmune diseases, such as rheumatoid arthritis or SLE

Pleurisy can also be a complication or side effect of chemotherapy, radiation, or surgery. Diagnosis is made based upon evaluation of symptoms, physical examination, and diagnostic imaging tests.

Treatment of pleurisy involves treating the underlying medical condition that's causing it, along with NSAIDs to relieve the pain and inflammation.

Pain in the Chest Wall

Costochondritis or Tietze's syndrome is the medical term for inflammation of the cartilage that joins the breastbone and the ribs. The costochondral joints are to blame. The pain can be sharp and severe and is felt in the area of the breastbone. If you press on this area, it feels painful. This condition is most common in adults between the ages of 20 and 40.

Upper respiratory viral infections and trauma may lead to costochondritis, and it's sometimes found in people with inflammatory bowel disease and certain autoimmune diseases, such as rheumatoid arthritis or SLE. It's also found in people who have had heart surgery. In many cases the cause can't be determined.

Diagnosis is based upon evaluation of symptoms and a physical examination that rules out other possible causes for the symptoms. Your physician may apply pressure to your skin over the area of the fourth to the sixth ribs. If this pressure is painful, it is a good diagnostic clue.

Treatment involves NSAIDs, and ice packs along with rest. That may mean stopping whatever the activity is that causes more pain until the symptoms have decreased. Gentle stretching of the pectoralis muscles may also prove helpful. In some cases, injection of corticosteroids to the affected area may be recommended. In most cases, costochondritis will get better on its own, and most patients report resolution of pain at about six months to a year.

Blockage of an Artery in the Lung

A blood clot in a lung artery is called a pulmonary embolism. The pain comes on abruptly and is sharp and severe. To some extent the symptoms mimic those of a heart attack, and they increase in severity when you cough (which may bring up blood) or take a deep breath. Other symptoms include anxiety and rapid heartbeat. A pulmonary embolism is an emergency situation and requires immediate medical care.

Risk factors include being inactive for extended periods of time, such as when traveling by plane or car or when confined to bed. Other risk factors include having had recent surgery or a fractured bone, using birth control pills or being pregnant, or having cancer.

Diagnosis is made based upon symptoms, physical examination, and diagnostic imaging tests of the lungs.

This pain is like that of a heart attack and can be a crushing, stabbing, shooting pain in the chest. It can cause severe feelings of oxygen hunger.

Treatment involves blood thinners (anticoagulants) such as heparin or Lovenox (enoxaparin), and after the clot has been dissolved, Coumadin (warfarin) to prevent further clots from developing.

Trauma

The internal organs of your chest, along with muscles and nerves and ligaments, are protected by your rib cage, an assemblage of bones and cartilage. Chest pain can result from strained muscles as well as from injury to the rib cage.

SPEAKING OF PAIN

Your 24 ribs actually belong to two of your body's systems: the skeletal and the respiratory systems. In addition to providing support, they expand and contract to allow your lungs to breathe.

Muscle Pain

Twisting while lifting can strain your chest muscles, and so can overexertion or participation in contact sports. The pain gets worse when you try to move from side to side or even when you try to take a deep breath.

Prevention involves paying attention to warm-ups and cool-downs, lifting heavy items by using your legs instead of your back, and engaging in regular, moderate exercise to strengthen muscles and increase flexibility.

Treatment involves NSAIDs, such as naproxen and ibuprofen, stretching, and application of cold. It may be difficult to remember to stretch an aching muscle, but in the end that may be the most beneficial therapy for you. Ask your doctor to recommend physical therapy for gentle stretching, and work with your physical therapist to get a good home regimen of stretching exercises for you to do.

Fractures

A fractured rib is an extremely painful injury. Because the ribs move each time you breathe, each breath you take hurts. A rib is considered fractured if there's a crack in it or if the bone is broken. Because the cartilage that attaches the ribs to the breastbone is so much a part of the rib cage, if part of this cartilage is ruptured, you're considered to have a fractured rib.

Accidents and falls are primary causes of fractured ribs, and any blow to the chest can result in a fracture. If you have osteoporosis or cancer, which can lead to thin and weakened bones, you can even fracture a rib by coughing.

It is possible to have other injuries in addition to the rib fracture, and your physician is the one to determine whether you've injured any internal organs in addition to your ribs.

The main symptom of a fractured rib is pain—pain when you breathe, pain when you move, and pain when any pressure is applied to your breastbone. Because of the pain, you may have trouble breathing and take more shallow breaths. Decreased oxygen supply can intensify feelings of anxiety.

Diagnosis is made based upon evaluation of symptoms, medical history, and a physical examination and x-rays. X-rays may be ordered to confirm the diagnosis, but these may be inconclusive. Your doctor may go on to order CT scans as well.

Unfortunately, the best treatment for a fractured rib is time, and rib fractures can take some time to heal. Most will heal on their own within 6 to 10 weeks.

Treatment for a fractured rib may include icing, rest, and NSAIDs. If the pain is severe, your physician may prescribe stronger pain medication. Taping isn't done anymore because it can interfere with deep breathing and increase your risk of pneumonia or a collapsed lung. You may find it easier to breathe if you lie on the side where the rib or ribs are broken.

Prevention of Chest Pain

For chest pain that's due to heart issues, reducing your risk of coronary artery disease is the best preventive strategy there is. This means not smoking, consuming only moderate amounts of alcohol, and observing a diet high in fiber and low in saturated fats. In addition, regular, moderate exercise can help you achieve and maintain a proper weight and lower your cholesterol. Your physician may prescribe that you take an aspirin each day to protect your heart.

If you engage in contact sports, be sure to wear protective gear to reduce your chances of rib injuries. Wearing your seat belt while driving and taking frequent breaks to get up and move around while traveling can reduce your chances of blood clots and prevent a possible pulmonary embolism.

Treatment

Treatment for pain associated with the heart can include both over-the-counter and prescription medications, such as NSAIDs, along with aspirin, nitroglycerin, beta blockers, calcium channel blockers, and other medications that work to keep blood from clotting.

Other options may include coronary bypass surgery and angioplasty.

Bruised, cracked, or broken ribs respond to rest and pain relievers. Time is what heals these injuries.

The Least You Need to Know

- Symptoms of a heart attack can vary widely. If you're having chest pain, get it checked out immediately.
- Cholesterol deposits in your arteries can cause a blockage that leads to heart attack or stroke.
- Exercise, not smoking, and eating a healthy diet can go a long way toward preventing heart disease and a heart attack.
- Deep breathing can help prevent lung collapse and pneumonia if you've fractured a rib.

Shoulder, Elbow, Wrist, and Hand Pain

In This Chapter

- When shoulder pain is an emergency
- Sports injuries
- Joint and tendon problems
- Repetitive motion and pain

Today's technology has given us a whole new range of painful maladies to supplement the age-old troubles of bursitis and tendonitis. Hours spent at a computer keyboard can result in days or weeks of pain in your wrist and finger joints. If you try to make up for a sedentary week with an overactive weekend, you risk injury to your shoulders, wrists, and elbows.

When to See the Doctor

Severe, sudden, crushing pain in your shoulder may be a symptom of a heart attack, especially if it radiates from your chest, jaw, or neck and down your arm and is accompanied by difficulty breathing, sweating, and/or dizziness. Call 911 for emergency medical assistance.

If you've been in an accident and incurred a blow to your shoulder, arm, wrist, or hand and you cannot use it, or if it appears deformed, swollen, is bleeding or badly bruised, you should seek immediate medical assistance.

Common sense should be your guide. If you've been self-medicating for what you believe to be a minor injury and it's not improving after two weeks, check with your doctor. This is especially important if you have other symptoms, such as a fever, which can indicate infection.

Diagnosis

Since injuries to these joints are fairly common, diagnosis is generally made based upon evaluation of your symptoms, analysis of your medical history, and a physical examination. Doctors can use diagnostic imaging tests to determine the specific point of injury or detect damage caused by a medical condition, such as osteoarthritis.

Sources of Shoulder Pain

Your shoulder is a ball and socket joint (like your hip), where the upper arm bone (called the humerus) attaches to the shoulder blade. The joint isn't especially deep, and this gives your arm a wide range of motion, allowing you to raise and lower it, move it from side to side, front to back, and swing it in an arc.

As with most aspects of life, there are tradeoffs. You have great flexibility and mobility with your shoulder, but because of the narrow placement of the humerus in the socket, it's not as stable as other ball and socket joints. The job of keeping your shoulder stable falls upon your rotator cuff, which is made up of four muscles and four tendons. An injury to your rotator cuff can definitely put you out of motion, and a few common injuries occur here.

Shoulder Tendinopathy

Tendons are tissues that attach muscles to bones. Tendinopathy is a general term that denotes injury to a tendon at the muscle-tendon unit. This injury can include inflammation in the tendon (called tendinitis) or microtears or tiny breaks in a tendon (called tendinosis). Rotator cuff tendinopathy and bicipital tendinopathy are two types of pain-causing problems in the shoulder.

The pain can occur through repetitive motion, overuse, or wear and tear that's a result of aging. Pain with throwing or reaching upward can occur and be worse during sleep. It can result in shoulder stiffness if the problem continues without treatment.

Diagnosis is made based upon symptoms, medical history, and a physical examination. During the exam, the doctor will check the range of motion and muscle strength of the affected area and will also look for tender areas. X-rays or an MRI may be advised to confirm the diagnosis.

Treatment consists of rest, along with alternating applications of ice and heat. Physical therapy, pain medications, nonsteroidal anti-inflammatory drugs (NSAIDs), and injection of a corticosteroid into the affected area may also be helpful. In severe cases, surgery may be necessary to correct the problem.

Bursitis

The fluid-filled sacs called bursae provide cushioning for tendons, muscles, and joints. In the shoulder, the bursae can become inflamed through repetitive motion, overuse, or trauma. This inflammation, called bursitis, is a common problem of shoulder joints and is usually brought on by overuse. Symptoms include pain when you move your shoulder, along with some swelling over the affected bursa. The area may also be painful to the touch.

Diagnosis is made based on symptoms, medical history, and a physical examination that includes a check of the range of motion of your shoulder and palpation for tenderness above the bursae. An MRI can be ordered to help confirm the diagnosis.

Treatment consists of rest, ice, physical therapy, and NSAIDs. Injection of a corticosteroid into the area may be helpful.

Rotator Cuff Injury

This painful injury is a common one among athletes and in adults after the age of 40. The rotator cuff is a group of muscles and tendons that cover the upper arm and allow it to rotate. This group of muscles and tendons can get injured in many ways.

Injuries include inflammation, microtears, complete tears, or a combination of these. For example, the tendon that attaches to the muscle on top of your shoulder (called the supraspinatus muscle) travels beneath the bone on the outside of your shoulder, a position that puts it between the bones of your shoulder joint. When you take a blow to your shoulder or have overused this joint, the tendon becomes inflamed or tears.

The resulting injury here is a sudden, sharp pain that can make it impossible for you to raise or rotate your arm. It can also make it difficult to bring your arm down when it is raised. Up or down, it doesn't matter. Your range of motion can be severely restricted.

The pain doesn't let up, and whenever you try to move the affected arm, you'll know that something is definitely wrong. If it's more than microtears or inflammation, the rotator cuff can actually tear. This can cause a snapping/popping feel or sound in the shoulder along with true weakness in which lifting the arm up above your head becomes impossible.

Diagnosis is made upon evaluating your symptoms and a physical examination, during which the doctor will test your range of motion in that arm. The pain is generally on the top and alongside your upper arm. The doctor can use diagnostic imaging tests to confirm a diagnosis. These tests include x-ray, arthrogram, arthroscopy, and ultrasound.

Treatment includes icing the shoulder, NSAIDs (ibuprofen, naproxen), use of a sling, possible injection of a corticosteroid, and *active rest*. The course of treatment depends on the type of injury that has occurred to the rotator cuff.

> **DEFINITION**
>
> **Active rest** is a balanced program of rest and mild low-impact aerobic exercise.

Your physician may refer you to physical therapy, where you'll learn how to exercise and strengthen the healing tendon and muscles. Your therapist will take you through a series of range-of-motion exercises, designed to stretch your shoulder, which will help it heal. As your shoulder improves, you'll learn specific resistance exercises that will continue to strengthen your shoulder.

In some cases, the tendon and muscle unit actually tears, and if physical therapy and medication aren't effective, you may need surgery to repair the damage.

Frozen Shoulder

The medical term for a frozen shoulder is *adhesive capsulitis*. There's nothing cold about this injury. The name refers to a painful condition in which your shoulder seems to be stuck and resists your efforts to move it. It's often a complication of a rotator cuff injury or of having not moved your shoulder normally for any reason, such as being in a sling after a fracture or being sick and lying in bed for a period of time. It can occur after a stroke when an arm is weak and mobility is compromised.

The onset of symptoms can be gradual or can progress quickly. Without intervention, you can suffer from this condition for a long time—even years.

SPEAKING OF PAIN

Most people who develop frozen shoulder are over the age of 40, and some statistics say that greater than 60 percent of them are women.

The tendons and ligaments in your shoulder are protected by a layer of connective tissue that encloses them. Sometimes this connective tissue thickens and tightens up, and the result is restricted motion for your shoulder. This condition progresses through three different stages:

1. The first stage is the painful one. It hurts to move your shoulder, and so you move it less and less as a result. The less you move your shoulder, the less it's able to move and your range of motion decreases. Often the pain gets worse at night.

2. The second stage is the one that gives its name to this condition. This is the frozen stage. It doesn't hurt as much, but your shoulder is noticeably stiff, and your range of motion decreases even more.

3. The third stage is called the thawing stage. Things gradually start to get better. The pain is generally gone; the stiffness begins to go away; and your range of motion increases again.

It's not clear just why this happens, although doctors suspect it may be an autoimmune response that develops after an injury to the shoulder and is more common in people with an underlying medical condition such as the following:

- Arthritis
- Stroke
- Diabetes
- Tuberculosis
- Recent surgery

Diagnosis is made based upon your symptoms, medical history, and a physical examination. Doctors may use diagnostic imaging tests to confirm the diagnosis.

Treatment includes NSAIDs, such as ibuprofen or naproxen, to reduce inflammation and relieve the pain. Injection of corticosteroids directly into the shoulder joint can also provide relief. Your physician may refer you to physical therapy for help in restoring motion to the shoulder. Range-of-motion exercises can be helpful for this condition. In some cases, surgery may be necessary to free up the shoulder joint.

Dislocation

This injury is the downside of the flexibility your shoulder has as a result of its being less stable than your other ball and socket joints. A dislocated shoulder is painful and requires immediate medical attention. It happens because the top of the arm bone (humerus) isn't firmly anchored in place; if it's hit with enough force, it can pop out of position.

You can dislocate your shoulder in a fall, if you're in an accident that delivers a hard blow to your shoulder, or if you participate in contact sports. It can also happen if you have a seizure or stroke. After your shoulder has been dislocated, there's a greater chance of it happening again. The more this happens, the more damage you can do to the ligaments and other tissue, and the weaker your shoulder can become.

Diagnosis is based upon your symptoms (which usually include a bump at the point of dislocation) and a physical examination. Diagnostic imaging tests may be used to rule out other causes of the pain (such as a broken bone).

Treatment involves manipulating the shoulder back into place. This procedure is called a closed reduction. Your physician will give you a sedative or a muscle relaxant before this procedure. She'll then gently move the shoulder back into its proper position. When the shoulder is back where it belongs, the intense pain should subside very quickly.

Your shoulder will need to be kept in place while the tissues heal, so you may need to wear a sling for a few weeks. Icing, along with NSAIDs, can help with pain relief. It can take several months for a dislocated shoulder to fully heal.

In some cases, surgery may be needed if your doctor can't return the joint to its proper position manually. This procedure is called an open reduction. Surgery may also be necessary if you've dislocated your shoulder more than once, as this can cause the tissues to weaken.

You may be referred to physical therapy to learn stretching and strengthening exercises to help strengthen the joint. Keeping this joint flexible can help prevent future injury.

STABS AND JABS

Trying to break a fall by using your hand can cause all kinds of problems, from a broken wrist to a separated or dislocated shoulder.

Shoulder Separation (AC Joint Separation)

Acromioclavicular (AC) separation can be confusing. The shoulder joint is made up of the clavicle (collarbone), shoulder blade (scapula) and the arm bone (humerus). The end of the scapula is called the acromion. The joint between the acromion and where the clavicle meets is called the AC joint. A result of the injury is a bump that usually develops at the point where the collarbone protrudes up toward the skin.

Separated shoulders can result from a fall, from an accident that delivers force to the shoulder, or from a contact sport. The pain is sudden and excruciating.

Diagnosis is made based upon symptoms and a physical examination. The telltale bump is good diagnostic information. Doctors may use diagnostic imaging tests to detect damage to other structures in the affected area.

Treatment includes icing, NSAIDs, and rest for your shoulder. Your physician may recommend a sling to help you keep your shoulder in place while the ligaments heal. In many cases the tendon will heal on its own, but if the tear is severe, surgery may be needed to repair the damage. This injury may take several weeks to heal. Not all shoulder separations are the same. Six subtypes of shoulder injury are classified based on the severity of the injury and how the bones are displaced. Some require surgery.

Your physician may also refer you to physical therapy to help strengthen the area and help protect against future injury. That bump is probably there to stay, although it won't hurt.

POINTERS ON PAIN

If you engage in contact sports, wear the proper protective equipment to protect your shoulders. Also, don't forget to warm up and cool down to help prevent injury.

Sources of Elbow Pain

Your elbow is a hinge joint, formed where your upper arm bone (humerus) joins up with the two bones of your lower arm (radius and ulna). This joint opens and closes like a hinge. When you extend your arm, the joint is fully open. When you bend your elbow and bring your wrist up toward your shoulder, the joint is closed. In addition to these motions, your elbow can also rotate, although not to the degree your shoulder can.

Trauma

Falls and accidents are the primary causes of fractures to the elbow. Fractures can occur either inside or just outside the joint. The elbow may appear misshapen, and pain can be severe.

Diagnosis is made based upon symptoms, a physical examination, and x-rays. Other diagnostic imaging tests can detect additional damage to soft tissues. Treatment requires casting; if the bones are severely damaged, orthopedic surgery may be necessary.

When the ligaments are ruptured or stretched, a sprain or strain results. Hyper-extension of the elbow happens when it incurs a force sufficient to cause it to bend opposite its natural design. This type of injury can result from a fall, contact sport, or accident. "Jamming" an elbow also causes stress upon the ligaments. Treatment includes icing, rest, compression, and NSAIDs.

Golfer's Elbow

The medical term for this condition is medial epicondylitis. This is an injury to the tendon that runs along the inside of your elbow and attaches to your forearm. A golf swing can cause this injury, but so can other activities that involve the same type of motion.

Golfer's elbow is painful. It's a tendon issue and not a joint problem, so it usually doesn't affect the range of motion of the joint. Usually it involves microtears and not inflammation, making the correct term "tendinosis" and not "tendinitis," which implies inflammation. The pain gets worse when you rotate your arm. It can be aggravated by carrying heavy items by the handles (such as paint cans or grocery bags) in your hands while your arms extend down by your sides. It can hurt to touch the affected area.

Golfer's elbow is diagnosed based upon your symptoms, medical history, and a physical examination that involves having you rotate your arm.

Treatment involves icing, rest, and NSAIDs. Remember, even if this problem is not due to inflammation, NSAIDs help with pain relief. Other medications for pain control such as acetaminophen can be just as effective. Injections of corticosteroids at the painful site can be helpful.

Tennis Elbow

The medical term for this condition is lateral epidoncylitis. This is tendinosis of the outside portion of the elbow, but you don't have to be a tennis player to sustain this injury. Again, this term (like medial epicondylitis) is misleading and can make you think inflammation is involved, but this isn't so. In reality, microtears occur in the tendon to cause this problem. Other than the result of numerous backhands, any repetitive forearm motion can cause it.

The outside of your forearm and elbow are painful and tender to the touch, but just as with golfer's elbow, it's a tendon issue, so your range of motion isn't affected. However, the more you use your arm, the more it hurts.

Tennis elbow is diagnosed based upon your symptoms, medical history, and a physical examination in which the doctor may apply slight pressure to your arm and ask you to move your arm.

Treatment involves icing, rest, and NSAIDs. Injection of corticosteroids into the affected area may be helpful.

Arthritis

When the elbow is inflamed and painful and injury has been ruled out, arthritis may be the source of the problem. Many times the problem is rheumatoid arthritis or another of the rheumatologic conditions, such as ankylosing spondylitis or gout. If an infection has occurred at the site, reactive arthritis may be the problem.

In addition to pain, inflammation causes decreased range of motion in your elbow. Treating the underlying condition may help restore your mobility with this joint. Over-the-counter or prescription NSAIDs may help relieve your symptoms.

Wrist pain can also be caused by arthritis. Osteoarthritis, the wear-and-tear variety of arthritis, can cause your wrists to hurt. The thumb is also often affected by osteoarthritis. In addition, other rheumatologic conditions, such as gout, ankylosing spondylitis, rheumatoid arthritis, or lupus, can cause wrist pain.

Funny Bone Pain

It's definitely a strange name for this condition, because there's nothing funny about the pain here. A nerve is responsible for this type of elbow pain. This nerve is the ulnar nerve, which runs from the tip of your elbow to the inner elbow bone. If you've banged your elbow, fallen, or been in an accident, this nerve can get pinched inside the bones. The resulting pain is burning and sharp. Often it can be due to resting your elbow while typing, or by driving for prolonged periods of time with your arms resting on the steering wheel. This condition is called ulnar nerve entrapment.

Other symptoms can include numbness and tingling in your hand, especially in your ring finger and pinkie. You might have some difficulty using the hand and find it's a bit awkward to manipulate.

Diagnosis is made based upon symptoms, medical history, and a physical examination, which may include the doctor asking you to raise your hand. This action may cause the numbness to return and is a helpful diagnostic clue. Other tests that can be done include electrodiagnostic testing.

Treatment involves bracing, icing, and NSAIDs for pain relief and to reduce swelling.

Sources of Wrist and Hand Pain

Your wrist is a complicated joint. In fact, it's not a single joint at all but is made up of a variety of smaller joints. This complexity is what gives it so much dexterity, agility, and capability.

Eight small carpal bones are in your wrist, and these small bones connect the larger bones of your forearm (radius and ulna) to the bones in your hand. The point where each of these bones attaches forms a joint, so the possibilities for hurting your wrist at a joint are numerous.

There's a considerable amount of symmetry between your hand and your foot, and the basic structures are the same. Your fingers, however, are a good deal longer than your toes, and that difference gives you all kinds of flexibility and dexterity.

Your hand is an intricate structure, made up of many bones, ligaments, tendons, and muscles—all enclosed in a fairly small space. There are 19 bones in your hand: 5 metacarpals extend from your wrist and across the center of your hand to your knuckles. The phalanges, 14 of them, form your fingers. Your thumb has 2 phalanges, and the rest of your fingers have 3 each. The place where phalange meets phalange forms a joint.

Trauma

Wrist injuries can be quite painful, and those injuries include fractures to the bones, sprains to the ligaments, or damage to the cartilage that serves as your joints' shock absorbers. Fractures to the wrist are often the result of falls or car accidents, especially when you try to break that fall with your hand or try to brace yourself by putting a hand on the glove compartment or dashboard before impact. Symptoms of a fracture may include a wrist that's obviously misshapen—sometimes with a portion of bone protruding through the skin—and difficulty moving the wrist, pain, bruising, and swelling. This type of injury requires medical attention.

Diagnosis

Diagnosis is based upon symptoms and a physical examination, along with diagnostic imaging tests. Treatment involves setting the broken bone and casting afterward to keep the wrist immobile while the bone heals. In some cases, surgery may be necessary to repair the damage.

Sprains or tears to the ligaments in the wrist are frequently the result of repetitive movements. If you've overused your wrist and sprained a ligament, it may feel sore and tender, but rest and icing will often take care of the problem.

If you've torn a ligament, however, the area may swell or appear bruised, and you may hear the characteristic popping or snapping sound when you try to use the wrist. Depending upon the severity of the tear, your physician may prescribe over-the-counter or prescription NSAIDs, along with icing, rest, and splinting. If the problem does not resolve, surgery may be necessary to repair the tendon.

Carpal Tunnel Syndrome

This is a term you're undoubtedly familiar with, and if you spend much time at the computer or at another activity that involves repetitive wrist motions, you may be familiar with the symptoms as well. In its early stages carpal tunnel syndrome can be an annoyance; however, as it progresses you may experience a chronic loss of feeling in some of your fingers, loss of strength in your wrist, and pain that doesn't get better when you stop using the wrist.

Carpal tunnel syndrome is a nerve injury that affects the median nerve in your wrist and/or palm. A narrow channel, called the carpal tunnel, in your wrist is designed to protect the median nerve, which fits nicely inside this channel.

With repetitive use of your wrist or for some other reason, the nerve can become inflamed and even severely injured. When this happens, it can swell and no longer fit nicely in the carpal tunnel. Instead, it's cramped, and it lets you know that it's cramped by sending a sharp, stabbing pain. The pain causes you to stop what's causing the irritation. Morning numbness and pain worse at that time is often a hallmark of the disease. When we sleep, the wrists are always flexed (that's our comfort position) and that tunnel physically gets smaller as we do. Instead of resting the wrist, our nighttime wrist position actually causes more compression and irritation.

Sometimes just stopping your motions momentarily helps, but other times it doesn't help at all, and the pain continues. Diagnosis of carpal tunnel syndrome is made based upon your symptoms, physical examination, and electrodiagnostic studies (see Chapter 4).

In addition to over-the-counter or prescription NSAIDs, your physician may prescribe a wrist brace to hold your wrist in a straighter position and keep it from moving about while the nerve heals.

De Quervain's Tenosynovitis (Mother's Wrist)

This condition is characterized by pain at the base or at the side of your thumb. The pain gets worse when you move the thumb in a variety of ways. Pinching motions, such as putting your thumb and index finger together, or pouring motions can aggravate the pain. Trying to unscrew a lid or turning a key—any motion that involves a turn of the wrist—can be painful.

You may find yourself dropping items because your thumb just doesn't want to cooperate. It's weak, and your hand can feel clumsy as a result. In fact, you may find it difficult to even make a fist. It's important to get treatment for de Quervain's tenosynovitis, because over time the pain can worsen, traveling up your arm and down your hand.

This is a tendon problem again and can be caused by inflammation, microtears of the tendon, or a combination of both. In fact, it's a "two-tendon" problem and involves the two main tendons of your wrist and thumb. Just as the nerve in your wrist travels through the carpal tunnel, the tendons also go through a small tunnel. When they become inflamed, there's just no room for them to maneuver.

De Quervain's tenosynovitis can be caused by overuse. That means it results from repetitive movements, such as those you may experience at work, doing certain household chores, or holding children, hence the name "mother's wrist." It can also be due to rheumatoid arthritis or trauma.

Treatment involves reducing the repetitive movements and resting your wrist. A brace can be helpful in keeping your wrist immobile while the inflammation subsides. Applying heat and taking NSAIDs can help relieve the pain and reduce the swelling.

If the condition doesn't improve within a few weeks, check with your doctor, as the longer this condition continues, the more chance of permanent damage to the tendons in your wrist. Injections of a corticosteroid around the tendon sheath can help reduce inflammation and speed recovery. In some cases surgery may be necessary.

The Least You Need to Know

- Never ignore pain that comes on suddenly and affects your shoulder or radiates to your arm or jaw. It could be a symptom of heart attack.
- A cramped nerve in the wrist is the source of carpal tunnel pain.
- Rotator cuff injuries are common and involve damage to one or more of the tendons that support your shoulder.
- A strain is an injury to a tendon or a ligament and often responds to rest and icing.
- Torn ligaments may require medical attention. A diagnostic clue is a characteristic popping or snapping sound.

Hip Pain

In This Chapter

- A common injury with life-threatening consequences
- Discovering the source of your hip pain
- Modern diagnostic procedures
- Preventing hip pain

Pain in your hip (or hips) can make walking, sitting, standing, and even lying down uncomfortable. As we age, wear and tear on this part of the body takes a serious toll; fractures in the elderly can be life-threatening. In this chapter, we'll cover the common causes of hip pain, as well as treatment options that provide welcome relief.

When to See the Doctor

There are levels of urgency in dealing with hip pain. Some hip pain constitutes an emergency situation and requires immediate medical attention. Generally such a condition occurs as a result of an accident or a fall. If you can't stand or put weight on your legs, or if there is bleeding, exposed tendons, or bone protruding through the skin, consider it a medical emergency. Call 911 for emergency assistance.

If your pain is severe and has come on suddenly, if your hip joint has swelled up or doesn't look "right" to you, if you recall hearing a snapping or popping sound at the time of injury, or if you've experienced loss of control over your bladder or bowels, don't wait to see whether these symptoms improve on their own. Have someone transport you to the emergency room for evaluation.

When you don't recall any trauma to your hip, and if the pain has come on gradually and there are signs of inflammation (such as tenderness, redness, and swelling, and if the area is warm to the touch), call your physician and schedule an appointment. In addition, call your physician if any of the following apply:

- You've been taking an over-the-counter pain medication for a week without any decrease in your pain.

- The pain is in both your hips (bilateral).

- You've been taking corticosteroids for an extended period of time.

- You've developed a fever or a rash.

Common sense needs to be your guide. Sometimes you're actually dealing with *referred pain*, which means the source of the pain is not your hip at all. Sometimes, even when the source of your pain is your hip, you may feel pain in your groin or along your thigh. Your physician is the one who can get to the crux of the problem.

DEFINITION

Referred pain occurs when you feel pain in one part of your body but the source is somewhere else. For example, pain associated with a heart attack may be felt in the left arm. This condition occurs because different nerve impulses are traveling along the same nerve pathway.

Diagnosis

If you've been transported to the emergency room, a triage nurse and then the emergency room physician will evaluate you. After an examination, you'll likely be sent to radiology for x-rays or other imaging tests.

If your hip pain is not an emergency and you've called your physician, you'll have an appointment scheduled. At that time, your physician will talk to you about your symptoms, review your medical history, and conduct a physical examination. Often the problem is fairly evident, especially if you're limping or using a cane or a walker and you report that you've fallen or injured your hip in some way.

Then diagnosis turns to determining how severe the injury is and what complications may be developing. In addition to asking you to stand, lie down, and walk, your doctor will conduct a hands-on examination of the painful area. X-rays and other imaging tests can help provide that information.

When injury isn't suspected as the cause of your hip pain, your doctor will begin ruling out certain medical conditions as the source. Blood work is the usual place to begin this process.

Diagnostic imaging, including x-ray and MRI with contrast material, is also indicated (see Chapter 4).

Arthrogram

Another imaging option is an arthrogram, which is the gold standard for diagnosing hip problems. For this procedure, which a radiologist usually performs, contrast material is injected into your hip joint and then x-rays are taken of the joint. The contrast material makes the soft tissues, such as muscles, ligaments, tendons, and cartilage, inside the joint clearly visible on the x-ray.

As with other diagnostic procedures that require a contrast material, tell your doctor whether you are pregnant or there is a possibility you may be pregnant.

In addition, tell your doctor if you have the following conditions:

- Diabetes
- Asthma
- Any infection in your hip
- Allergies to contrast materials (these may include dyes or iodine)
- Allergies to anesthetics
- Allergies to any medicines
- Allergies to shellfish

If you are taking blood thinners, are currently experiencing a flare-up of your arthritis, have ever had any type of allergic reaction (such as sensitivity to bee stings), or have had any previous reactions to a diagnostic procedure, let your physician know before you have an arthrogram.

For the procedure, you will lie down on the exam table. A nurse or technician will clean the skin above your hip with an antiseptic solution. After that, you'll be given a local anesthetic to numb the area where the needle will be inserted.

You will be awake for the procedure so that you'll be able to move if the radiologist wants to get a different angle for the pictures or if he wants the dye (sometimes air is used for this purpose) to spread to a different location in your hip.

When the needle is inserted you may feel a pinch, and sometimes the anesthetic stings a bit as it's injected. If air is used, you may feel some pressure in your hip; if dye is used, it may sting. The entire procedure takes anywhere from half an hour to an hour, depending upon what the doctor is looking for and what he finds after he can see inside the joint space.

After the arthrogram is finished, you're free to go. You'll be given instructions to rest that joint for a specific length of time—usually the rest of the day. If the injection site is sore, you can apply ice to reduce any swelling. Over-the-counter pain medication can help ease any residual discomfort, which should go away within a day or so.

POINTERS ON PAIN

What's all the noise? After an arthrogram it takes a while for the air or liquid that was injected into the joint to dissipate. In the meantime, that clicking and crackling sound will be your personal percussion section.

Arthroscopy

Diagnosis may also require arthroscopy of the hip joint. You can read about arthroscopy as a surgical procedure in Chapter 9. As a diagnostic procedure, however, arthroscopy allows your physician to look inside your hip joint and assess the damage.

She'll make a small incision in the skin and insert the arthroscope, a tiny tubelike instrument equipped with optical lenses, fibers, and a video camera to take pictures of the interior of your hip. You can watch the progress on a computer screen.

Sources of Hip Pain

Hip pain can have many sources, including injury, infection, and overuse. In some cases, the pain is a symptom of an underlying medical condition.

The hip is a ball and socket type of joint. It's formed where the thigh bone from your upper leg (the ball part of the joint) meets your pelvis (the socket part of the joint). In addition to these bones, this site also has cartilage, muscle, and other soft tissue—each of which can be a source of pain.

Fracture

This is the most common type of hip injury in older people, and specifically in women after the age of 65. A fractured pelvis presents with symptoms similar to those with a fractured hip.

It usually isn't the entire joint that breaks, but rather the upper portion of the femur (the ball part of the socket).

Often these fractures are the result of advanced osteoporosis (thinning of the bones), which can make a simple fall or bump life-threatening. In addition, many elderly people have poor balance, which contributes to the risk for fractures.

Complications are a serious consequence of some hip fractures because the patient is unable to move about. A blood clot in the leg is a potential complication because it can migrate to the lungs, where it can be fatal. Pneumonia is another concern.

 SPEAKING OF PAIN

Hip fractures are serious injuries. Fewer than 50 percent of people who fracture a hip are able to return to their previous activity level.

Surgery is generally indicated to repair a hip or pelvic fracture caused by impact injury.

Strains and Sprains and Bruises

You generally think of ankles when you think sprains, but it's possible to sprain your hip. A sprained hip is a ligament injury. A strained hip occurs when you injure one of the muscles or tendons associated with your hip.

Usually these injuries happen when you're twisting while lifting, as the result of an accident, or simply from putting too much load on your hips. The muscles, tendons, and ligaments become inflamed, and inflammation hurts.

A bruised hip is generally the result of a fall or other accident. If you're carrying items in your arms and your vision is blocked, it's entirely possible to walk into a door or other piece of furniture with enough force to bruise your hip.

Hip Pointer

This type of hip injury is almost a badge of honor. It says you're an athlete, or at least you're exercising like one. This injury is nothing to laugh about, however. It's extremely painful.

A hip pointer results when the *iliac crest* of the pelvis sustains a trauma, usually the result of a serious fall or a direct blow. You don't have to be an athlete to get it. The bone can be bruised, along with the surrounding muscles. If you play any contact sports, such as football, soccer, or rugby, you're probably familiar with this type of injury.

 DEFINITION

The **iliac crest** is the rim of the ilium, the big bone located at the upper portion of the pelvis. You can feel the iliac crest with your hands when you press in along your sides just below the waist.

Symptoms include acute pain that's felt with walking, coughing, or laughing, and even deep breaths can be excruciating.

Rest is the usual method of treatment, coupled with over-the-counter pain relievers. Wearing the correct protective athletic pads can help prevent hip pointers.

Dislocation

A dislocation occurs when the femur is forced away from the pelvic socket. It is an extremely painful injury and most often occurs as the result of an accident or fall from a considerable height, such as down the stairs.

Dislocation is a medical emergency and requires immediate treatment. Call 911 and do not move the person. At the emergency room, diagnosis is fairly straightforward, because the leg is at an unnatural angle.

Treatment involves using an anesthetic or a sedative before manipulating the femur by hand to return it to the socket. Sometimes surgery is required to repair a dislocated hip.

In most cases the dislocation heals within a few months, but complications can occur with a dislocation. These include nerve damage and damage to the cartilage. If the blood supply to the bone is interrupted, the bone can actually die, a condition called osteonecrosis (osteo = bone, necrosis = death). If this occurs, hip replacement surgery may be necessary immediately.

Bursitis

Bursae are fluid-filled little pouches that work like cushions near your joints. They keep the muscles, tendons, and bones from rubbing together and function in a way similar to cartilage.

Sometimes, when you've overused the joint, these bursae get irritated and inflamed. Overuse can actually seem like no use at all, when you're talking about your hips. Sitting for extended periods of time can cause the bursae around your hip to scream for help. Symptoms include painful movement and even pain when you touch the joint, which can also feel stiff.

Diagnosis is usually made by evaluating your symptoms, although if injury can't be verified, your doctor may order imaging tests. Imaging tests will also help to rule out the possibility of another medical condition as the cause of your bursitis pain.

In most cases, rest and over-the-counter pain relievers such as ibuprofen or naproxen will be effective in treating bursitis.

Snapping Hip Syndrome

This may sound like some sort of strange dance step, and in fact this condition is often referred to as "dancer's hip." It's an audible condition; when you move your hips, you can hear a snapping or popping sound. The sound is most often caused by tendons temporarily getting hung up on bone and then snapping back into position.

Two specific tendons are involved. The first one (called the iliotibial band) is on the outside of the hip joint. When this tendon irritates the neighboring bursae, you can develop a painful case of bursitis.

The second tendon (called the iliopsoas tendon) is located right in front of the hip joint. This condition is not usually painful, but the noise can be distracting.

POINTERS ON PAIN

In some cases, torn cartilage inside the hip joint can result in snapping hip syndrome. This is called a hip labral tear and can be quite painful.

Diagnosis is generally made by evaluating the symptoms. Imaging tests may be used to be sure there are no additional injuries to the area.

Pain relief can usually be obtained with over-the-counter anti-inflammatory medications, such as ibuprofen or naproxen. A cortisone injection may also be prescribed if the pain is ongoing or severe. To prevent future problems, your physician may recommend physical therapy to strengthen muscles and stretch ligaments.

Impingement Syndrome

You want the femur to fit snugly in the pelvic socket. If it's too loose, you run the risk of dislocation; if it's too tight, the head of the femur rubs against the pelvic socket. When this happens, because the femur is "over-covered" by the socket, it's called impingement syndrome. Impingement syndrome is a condition in which the femur grinds away at the bone, causing torn ligaments, bone spurs, and pain.

Diagnosis is made by evaluating your symptoms and using imaging tests to pinpoint the problem. It's important to treat this condition early, so it doesn't develop into arthritis. Anti-inflammatory medications can help with pain relief. New procedures using arthroscopic surgery techniques can remove the excess bone and bone spurs and repair torn ligaments.

Infection

Bacteria and viruses can lead to infection in your hip. Because infection comes with inflammation, your pain can be quite intense. Specific infections include the following:

- Reactive arthritis (a type of arthritis that can develop after an intestinal or urinary tract infection)

- Septic or infectious arthritis (resulting from a bacterial infection in the hip)

- Lyme disease (transmitted through a tick bite)

- Food poisoning

- Infection as a complication of surgery

Diagnosis is usually made through blood work analysis and imaging tests. Treatment is with antibiotics.

Muscle Tightness

The muscles in your groin are responsible for keeping your leg in proper alignment. These five muscles are called the adductor muscles. These muscles also help you move your hip. They can become injured when you move abruptly from one position to another, putting strain on them.

Tightness can occur from injury, overuse, or improper use. It's important to warm up before exercising and use the right muscle group for whatever job you have in mind.

Treatment involves rest, icing, anti-inflammatory medications, and physical therapy.

> **POINTERS ON PAIN**
>
> Referred hip pain can come from a hernia, radiculpathy (pinched nerve), or an underlying medical condition, such as diabetes.

Osteoarthritis

Hip pain is a symptom of many medical conditions, and osteoarthritis is the first one that comes to mind. Thanks to advances in medical science and nutrition, we're living longer. That's good news, of course, but it also means that we're making more demands on our body's joints, and our hips carry their fair share of the load.

Osteoarthritis is the wear-and-tear form of arthritis and is a principal reason for hip replacement surgeries, which are becoming increasingly common. There are several risk factors for developing osteoarthritis, including having a member of your family with osteoarthritis, as there seems to be a genetic component for this disease.

Additional risk factors include being obese, elderly, or having had a previous injury to your hips. Sometimes, you may not have any identifiable risk factors but develop this condition anyway.

> **SPEAKING OF PAIN**
>
> It is estimated that more than 10 million Americans have osteoarthritis.

Symptoms of hip osteoarthritis may start as some stiffness and general soreness in your groin, buttock, or thigh area upon waking. This feeling usually improves as the day progresses and you go about your routine. Gradually, however, this condition doesn't improve as the day goes on. The stiffness and soreness seem to have settled in for the duration, and resting doesn't help.

What's happening is that the bones in your hip joint have lost their cartilage insulation, and they're constantly grating against each other with every move you make. Bone spurs can develop around the joint, which is now inflamed.

The next phase will find you unable to move your hip joint through its normal range of motion. Extending, flexing, and rotating are no longer possible. Since the muscles supporting the joint aren't getting any exercise, they lose tone and can't do their jobs.

Walking or any movement that involves your hips, even standing and getting up out of a chair, is now painful, and you are probably limping. Hopefully you've seen a doctor long before the osteoarthritis has progressed to this point. Early diagnosis and treatment can prevent a great deal of pain and disability, along with the need for surgery.

Diagnosis includes a physical examination, medical history evaluation, and diagnostic imaging of the hips.

Treatment options at the early stage include losing extra weight, therapeutic rest and exercise, physical therapy, and nonsteroidal anti-inflammatory drugs (NSAIDs). In more advanced cases, hip replacement surgery may be necessary.

Other Medical Conditions

Sometimes there's no obvious reason for your hip pain, and finding the exact cause takes careful diagnostic work. Other medical conditions that can include hip pain as a symptom are as follows:

- Other forms of arthritis, including psoriatic and rheumatoid
- Cancers, including bone cancer and leukemia
- Lupus
- Hemophilia
- Rheumatic fever
- Shingles
- Sickle cell disease
- Bone disorders, including osteomalacia, osteomyelitis, and osteochondromatosis

- Spinal stenosis

- Paget's disease

- Nerve injury

Only your physician can determine whether any of these conditions are responsible for your hip pain. Treating the condition can help relieve pain that centers around your hips.

Prevention

Much hip pain can be prevented, and prevention is definitely preferable to having to repair the damage with surgery. Many instances of hip pain occur as the result of trauma, so taking precautions to reduce your risk for accidents is definitely recommended.

It's often when you let safety slide that you get hurt. Simple steps to prevent injury to your hips include always buckling up when you get in the car. Automobile accidents are a main cause of hip fractures.

 STABS AND JABS

Falls can be deadly. Especially as you age, take precautions to safeguard yourself. Take up any small scatter rugs. These can become "flying carpets," and you'll have a hard landing.

Place adhesive no-skid strips on stairs to give you good traction and prevent slips. These are available at hardware stores. They usually come on a roll, enabling you to cut a strip to the right length to fit on each stair.

Kitchen chairs tip over easily. Use a step ladder instead of a kitchen chair when you need to reach something above your head. And don't stand on the step above the safety level. You'll find this point marked on all ladders. A reach extender is a lifesaver, especially when you're trying to get at something on a top shelf.

Keeping fit is your best safeguard for hip health. Exercise and good nutrition are your best friends for life. Take time to stretch and warm up before engaging in vigorous exercise. Avoid jerking movements that put stress and strain on your hips. Exercise regularly. Manage your weight. Being overweight puts you at increased risk for hip injuries and for developing osteoarthritis in your hips.

Treatment

Because there are so many causes of hip pain, treatment involves addressing the medical issue that's the source of your pain.

If you have a medical condition such as diabetes, arthritis, sickle cell anemia, or any others listed in the previous section, be sure your treatment is up-to-date and that you're managing your symptoms in the best way possible.

Seek treatment earlier rather than later. If your over-the-counter pain relievers aren't helping your hip pain after a week, schedule an appointment with your physician to find out what the problem is and the best way to treat it.

If you don't know why your hip is hurting or if you've been in an accident, don't take chances. Call your doctor and find out what to do.

NSAIDs such as ibuprofen or naproxen can help relieve hip pain caused by inflammation that's a result of arthritis, bursitis, or tendinitis.

Your doctor may refer you to physical therapy to get you back on track. A program of regular exercise that includes low-impact aerobic activity (such as walking, swimming, or cycling) can strengthen the muscles supporting your hip joint, which will help you move with less pain.

The Least You Need to Know

- A fractured hip is a medical emergency. Call 911.
- Minor hip injuries usually respond well to rest and over-the-counter pain medication.
- Accidents and falls are the major causes of hip injuries. Practice prevention.
- Physical therapy can strengthen the muscles that support your hip joint to reduce pain and increase fitness.

Knee, Shin, and Foot Pain

In This Chapter

- Common knee injuries
- Overuse problems with your legs
- Taking care of your feet and ankles
- Prevention is key

Your knees are your body's workhorses, and your feet and ankles take you where you want to go. They allow you to walk, run, and jump, and they support you when you stand. As with your hips, your knees may eventually simply wear out. When they are causing you pain, there are ways to get relief. In this chapter, we'll show you how.

When to See the Doctor

Sprains and strains generally respond well to rest, icing, and over-the-counter anti-inflammatory medications, but knowing the difference between a mild sprain and a torn ligament or a bruised instep from a stress fracture requires the professional expertise of your physician.

If your knee, ankle, or foot is noticeably swollen, changed in shape, warm to the touch, or inflamed, or if you can't bear weight on it, it's best to have it checked out. And if you're running a fever, along with pain in any of your joints, an infection may be the culprit, and your doctor is the one to treat the problem.

Treating problems in this area sooner rather than later can save you a considerable amount of potential future discomfort and help you continue with your normal daily activities. When pain forces you to change the way you walk, you put strain on your hips and back. It doesn't take long for muscles, tendons, ligaments, and discs to rebel at being misused. Then you'll have more pain issues to address. Being proactive can head off many serious problems in these areas.

Diagnosis

An evaluation of your symptoms, your medical history, and a physical examination will often provide your doctor with enough information to make a diagnosis. To check for knee injuries, such as torn ligaments, the doctor will look for signs of swelling or tenderness and check your range of motion.

POINTERS ON PAIN

Every joint has a normal range in which it moves and is supposed to move without difficulty. Often with pain, swelling, or other injuries, this normal arc of movement can be compromised.

If your foot is the problem, the doctor will physically manipulate the structures of your foot by rotating your ankle, flexing your arch, or applying resistance to the sole. Your doctor might also use touch, ice, or perhaps a cotton swab during the foot exam.

Finding the spot or areas that cause pain is also part of the process. You may be asked to stand and/or walk (on your toes or heels). In some cases, and especially if there is a great deal of swelling that prevents a good check of range of motion, diagnostic imaging tests will be ordered to see whether there is damage to bone or soft tissues.

Blood work may be ordered to rule out infection or one of the arthritic conditions, such as gout, as the source of your pain.

Sources of Knee Pain

Your knee is a rather complicated *hinge joint*, made up of four bones tied together by four ligaments. These bones include the femur (thighbone) from your upper leg, the tibia and fibula (shinbone) from your lower leg, and the patella (kneecap). To support your knee and protect it from injury, ligaments run along the inside and outside of the knee and also form an "X" as they crisscross from the end of your femur to the top of your shinbone.

DEFINITION

A **hinge joint** gets its name because it opens and closes just like a door hinge. The knee is one of your body's biggest and heaviest hinge joints. It's also capable of slight rotating and twisting movements.

In addition to the bones and ligaments, your knee also houses two tendons that join muscle to bone, the meniscus (cartilage), and some bursae (fluid-filled sacs) that provide cushioning. That's quite a bit of equipment concentrated in a small space, so it's not surprising that pain can be a frequent visitor to your knees.

Many knee and ankle injuries are sports-related. Whether the result of direct contact with another player, the ground, or other hard surface, or simply from repetitive use, this part of the body takes more than its share of abuse. Sometimes just landing wrong after jumping or quick turns or pivots can cause problems.

Dislocated Kneecap

Generally the result of a sideways blow to the knee, this type of injury causes the patella (kneecap) to move out of position, generally toward the outside of the knee. Once out of place it tends to move around quite a bit. A dislocated kneecap is extremely painful and is accompanied by swelling. You may find it impossible to put weight on that leg or straighten your knee.

Hyperextension

This injury occurs when your knee has reached its maximum degree of extension, which means it's essentially straight up and down. A blow of some type to the knee causes the knee joint to bend the opposite way it was intended to operate. It essentially bends backward. It's painful, and if the blow is severe enough and the knee hyper-extends too much, you can tear a ligament. The most commonly affected ligament with this injury is the anterior cruciate ligament (ACL).

SPEAKING OF PAIN

Each year, more than 30 percent of the American population above the age of 45 have knee pain of some sort.

Cartilage Tears

The cartilage inside your knee joint is called the meniscus. Tears in the meniscus are accompanied by swelling that may not begin immediately after you've injured your knee, but may take a day or two to become noticeable. You probably won't be able to straighten your knee, and you'll feel quite a bit of pain with this injury.

Ligament Injuries

Any of the four ligaments inside your knee can be torn as the result of a direct blow or a fall. The pain comes on quickly and gets worse if you try to bend or put any weight on your knee. There may be a popping noise when you move your knee.

Bursitis

When the bursae that cushion your knee become inflamed, you may find that your knee hurts when you go up and down stairs or when you kneel. Walking can be painful, and your knee may feel stiff. In addition, your knee may feel warm to the touch and be swollen. It may hurt even when you're not using it.

Tendinitis

Inflammation of the tendon that connects the quadriceps thigh muscle with the shinbone is a common sports-related injury for cyclists, skiers, and runners. It is also called Jumper's knee. You may find your range of motion affected to the point that you can't fully straighten your leg. In addition to pain in your knee, there may be swelling across the front or below. Any movement that puts strain on that tendon (such as jumping, kneeling, or climbing stairs) causes the symptoms to get worse.

POINTERS ON PAIN

Those popping sounds coming from your knee could be the sound of tendons rubbing over bones in the joint (usually not painful or harmful) or could be a sign of dislocation, especially if you heard a pop at the time of an injury to the knee (painful!).

Iliotibial Band Syndrome

This is a fairly common knee injury, especially among distance runners. The ligament that extends from your hip across your kneecap and down your shin is called the iliotibial band. With repetitive knee flexing and extending, this band can become inflamed and tighten up as it passes over the thighbone.

The pain with this injury can be sharp and burning and is situated on the outer side of the knee and thigh. Early on it tends to get better with rest, but if the overuse continues, the pain may become constant. For athletes, cutting back on training can give the band time to rest and relax.

Physical therapy that works on stretching the iliotibial band and strengthening the hip abductor muscles and stretching the adductors is often used to treat iliotibial band syndrome. If it doesn't respond to therapy, injections of corticosteroids or even surgery may be necessary.

Baker's Cyst

A Baker's cyst, sometimes also called a popliteal cyst, generally develops as a result of an underlying medical condition, such as arthritis or a tear in the kneecap's cartilage—conditions that cause your knee to produce too much fluid. Symptoms include a bulging and feeling of tightness in back of the knee, as if the skin is being stretched. Trying to straighten your knee makes the pain worse.

These cysts generally go away on their own after the condition that caused them has been treated. If they are causing discomfort, the fluid can be drained, or they can be surgically removed if necessary.

POINTERS ON PAIN

P.R.I.C.E. stands for Protection, Rest, Ice, Compression, and Elevation—important procedures for treating injuries to this portion of your body.

Arthritis

Osteoarthritis is a common cause of knee pain, particularly in older adults, and it's a main reason for knee replacement surgeries. In addition to this wear-and-tear type of arthritis, rheumatoid arthritis can cause knee pain as well.

Other rheumatologic conditions that can cause knee pain include septic arthritis that develops as the result of an infection, gout, or pseudogout. (See *The Complete Idiot's Guide to Arthritis* for a complete discussion of these conditions, including diagnosis and treatment.)

Treatment for arthritis of the knee includes rest, physical therapy, nonsteroidal anti-inflammatory drugs (NSAIDs), and in severe cases, surgery.

Sources of Shin Pain

In addition to fractures, bruises, and scrapes, your shin can become sore as the result of what's commonly called "shin splints." Shin splints can result from overusing this part of your leg, and this condition is common in runners and power walkers.

Problems with your Achilles tendon or your ankles can also contribute to your developing shin splints. A well-known cause of people getting shin splints is flat feet.

Characteristically, athletes will feel pain as they begin their workouts. This pain decreases during the activity but then returns at the end. It often starts as a dull ache and progresses to a sharp pain that can interfere with practice to the point that any use becomes impossible.

Diagnosis of shin splints is made with a review of symptoms and a physical examination. If a stress fracture is suspected, x-rays may be used to confirm the diagnosis.

Treatment includes resting the leg, along with icing. Stretching and strengthening exercises can help with both treatment and prevention of future problems in this area.

Sources of Ankle or Foot Pain

Just like your knee, your ankle is a hinge joint, although it's capable of quite a bit more variety with regard to movement. You can rotate your ankle and flex it from side to side with a much greater range of motion than with your knee. The ankle consists of your ankle bone and the ends of your shinbone (the tibia and fibula). Ligaments tie these bones together. Tendons, which attach the muscles to the bones, along with those muscles, provide additional strength and mobility.

Falls are the biggest danger to ankles and, depending upon how you land, you may incur a sprain (injury to a ligament), a fracture (broken bone), or an injury to the tendon, muscle, or cartilage.

POINTERS ON PAIN

The term "sprain" is often a misnomer. Often sprain implies that inflammation is present, but it also means that there are micro-tears in the ligament.

If you've fallen or been in an accident and notice swelling and acute pain that prevent you from putting any weight on the ankle, you may have a fracture or a severe sprain. If your ankle is bruised with some swelling but you can still walk on it, it may be sprained, or you may have a fracture of the smaller shinbone (fibula).

Pain that comes on without prior trauma may indicate an infection, especially if you're running a fever. Patients who are diabetic need to be aware of this possibility with regard to the ankle and knee joints. Other sources of ankle pain include osteo-arthritis or other rheumatologic conditions, such as rheumatoid arthritis or gout.

STABS AND JABS

If both of your ankles are swollen and you're running a fever, call your doctor. These could be symptoms of rheumatic fever.

Sources of Foot Pain

Your foot is surprisingly strong, and it needs to be to carry your body's weight and transport you where you wish to go. With 24 bones; more than 30 joints; 2 arches; and more than 120 muscles, nerves, and ligaments, each foot is a complex structure with many opportunities for injury to create some painful situations.

In addition to injury, certain medical conditions, such as diabetes, pregnancy, or obesity, can create painful foot problems.

Achilles Tendonitis

Your body's biggest and strongest tendon, called the Achilles tendon, extends down the back of your lower leg and attaches your leg muscles to your foot at the heel. When this tendon becomes inflamed, you not only feel sharp pain, but you may find it impossible to walk or even flex your toes. It can be an incapacitating condition.

Achilles tendonitis can be triggered by sudden changes in movement or in the intensity of that movement. For example, breaking into a run from a dead stop, instead of warming up first, can cause the tendon to become inflamed.

STABS AND JABS

Wearing high-heeled shoes can shorten your Achilles tendon over time. When you change to flat-heeled shoes, your tendon must stretch beyond its accustomed length, inviting injury.

This injury can be diagnosed by evaluating your symptoms and a good physical examination. A test that a doctor can do in the office is called the Thompson test. It can be done to determine whether you've ruptured the tendon. You'll lie face down on the exam table and bend your knees at a 90-degree angle so that your feet are parallel with the ceiling. The doctor will squeeze your calf to see whether there's any movement in your ankle. If there isn't, you've probably torn it.

Your doctor can use diagnostic imaging tests, such as ultrasound or an MRI, to confirm a diagnosis. Treatment for minor Achilles tendon injuries involves rest, anti-inflammatory medications, such as naproxen or ibuprofen, icing, elevating the foot to reduce swelling, and physical therapy. Patients with flat feet will also stretch their Achilles tendon if they wear proper orthotics (shoe inserts designed to take pressure off certain areas). In severe injuries, surgery may be necessary to reattach the tendon.

Blisters

Blisters are caused by rubbing, and in the case of your feet, this rubbing generally results from ill-fitting shoes. The area becomes tender and can begin to burn. If the rubbing continues, the area becomes sore, and fluid accumulates under the skin, forming a blister.

If the blister pops and the fluid drains, cover the area with a sterile bandage to help prevent infection. Protect the skin from further damage while it's healing with a gel pad or donut. Address the problem that's causing the blister, and you won't get a repeat performance.

Puncture Wounds

Puncture wounds from nails or other sharp objects generally occur on the bottom of the foot and can quickly become infected. It's important to keep current on your tetanus shot to protect against this serious complication of puncture wounds. If you are diabetic, appropriately treating the puncture wound is even more important as diabetes slows the healing process.

Turf Toe

This injury gets its name from the playing surface of football, soccer, baseball, and rugby fields. A contact injury, this happens when the tendon under the big toe is strained and becomes inflamed.

Diagnosis is made based on symptoms and medical history. If necessary, x-rays or an MRI can be done to confirm the diagnosis.

Treatment consists of rest, icing, compression, and elevation. Wearing the proper footwear for the activity can help with prevention of turf toe.

Inflammation of the Ball of the Foot

This condition, called sesamoiditis, refers to inflammation of the tendons attached to the sesamoid bones in the ball of your foot close to your big toe. High-impact aerobics and jogging can put excessive stress on these tendons, resulting in strain.

Diagnosis is made based on symptoms and physical examination. X-rays may be used to confirm the diagnosis. Backing off on exercise and resting the ball of your foot frequently are all that's needed to give the tendons time to recuperate. In some cases, an injection of a corticosteroid into the affected area may be helpful. In severe cases, surgery may be required to repair the damage.

Morton's Neuroma

The name may sound exotic, but Morton's neuroma is a fairly straightforward condition. Simply put, the tissue around the nerves that lead to your toes can thicken. This then causes the bones of your third and fourth toes to close ranks, and a nerve gets compressed in the process. The nerve becomes inflamed and swells. You may feel cramping on the topside of your foot, along with a burning sensation (a classic symptom of nerve damage).

Diagnosis is made based upon symptoms and a physical examination. Ultrasound or an MRI can be used to confirm the diagnosis.

Culprits here are ill-fitting shoes, congenital foot problems, arthritis, or trauma to the top of the foot. Treatment involves massage, better-fitting shoes, and maybe injections to help decrease pain. In severe cases that don't respond to these measures, surgery is given as an option.

Stress Fracture

This injury, also referred to as a fatigue fracture, occurs when one of the *metatarsal bones* of the foot is ruptured or broken. Usually the second or third metatarsals are more prone to this type of injury. The metatarsal leading to your big toe is much thicker than the other metatarsals and is more resistant to this injury. If it is fractured, however, this injury can be more serious than a fracture in the thinner metatarsals.

DEFINITION

The **metatarsal bones** are the long bones in your foot that extend from your ankle to the bases of your toes.

Stress fractures are usually considered to be "overuse" injuries and occur when you put too many demands on your feet.

Diagnosis is made based upon symptoms, physical examination, and medical history. In some cases, a bone scan or ultrasound may be used to confirm a diagnosis and assess the extent of the damage.

Stress fractures generally heal by themselves within a few weeks, if you rest your foot and wear low-heeled shoes. If the pain continues after three weeks, surgery may be needed to correct the condition.

Tarsal Tunnel Syndrome

This condition is essentially carpal tunnel syndrome of the foot. A tunnel extends from behind your inner ankle bone to your heel. This tunnel provides the housing for a nerve called the tibial nerve. When that nerve is compressed because of injury, the result is pain and numbness of the foot and toes.

Tarsal tunnel syndrome can have a variety of causes, including diabetes, arthritis, trauma to the ankle, scar tissue around the nerve, or blood vessel irregularities.

Diagnosis is based upon symptoms, physical examination, and diagnostic imaging tests, including an MRI. Treatment may include orthotics, injections of corticosteroids, and in severe cases, surgery.

Arch Pain

Your foot has two arches. The arch that extends along the sole of your foot is called the longitudinal arch, and the one that extends across your foot is called the transverse arch. These arches are tied together with ligaments, supported by muscles and tendons, and cushioned by fat pads. A problem with any of these components can cause arch pain.

Diagnosis of arch pain is made by evaluating symptoms, a physical examination, and diagnostic imaging tests.

Treatment may consist of NSAIDs, rest, and stretching exercises. Shoe inserts (orthotics) may be helpful in relieving pain.

Plantar Fascia (Plantar Fasciitis)

Though the term "fasciitis" implies that inflammation is the cause of the problem, this is incorrect. Plantar fasciitis is caused by degeneration of the thick fibrous band that is attached to the heel bone and fans out to the entire foot. This is a common cause of heel pain. The pain intensity generally follows an arc pattern. If you've been asleep or resting and then stand, you may notice pain in your heel. After you begin walking or exercising, the pain decreases, only to increase again after you've been at your activities for some time.

During rest, the muscles in your foot tighten up, which strains the plantar fascia. Exercise stretches the muscles, but extended exercise causes inflammation, and the pain returns. Your heel may feel warm to the touch and may appear red—both signs of inflammation.

Plantar fasciitis often stems from an arch problem—your arches may be too high or too low (flat feet). It can also be caused by—yep, you guessed it—ill-fitting shoes. If your work requires you to be standing for long periods of time on hard surfaces, such as concrete, you need shoes that support your arches.

POINTERS ON PAIN

Flat feet, also known as *pes planus* or fallen arches, can be a painful condition. Arch inserts in your shoes can help relieve this pain, but sometimes medication or even surgery is necessary to correct the problem.

Being overweight is also a contributing factor in developing plantar fasciitis. Also, if you are unable to stretch or use the dorsiflexor muscles of the leg (the muscles in your leg that bring your toes up toward your shin), then plantar fasciitis may be in your future. Patients who wear high heels, runners, and flat-footed people are all at potential risk for this condition.

Diagnosis is made through an evaluation of symptoms and a physical examination. Diagnostic imaging tests may be ordered to rule out other heel conditions.

Treatment options include the following:

- Icing

- Physical therapy and stretching exercises

- Footwear that supports your arches

- NSAIDs, such as naproxen and ibuprofen

- A walking cast that you can remove when you're at rest

- Injections of corticosteroids

Additionally, if you are overweight, losing that extra weight will take strain off your plantar fascia. In some cases, surgery may be required to correct this condition.

Bunions

You're probably quite familiar with the outward appearance of this common foot condition. The classic presentation is a large bony bump at the outside of the base of the big toe. The toe then angles inward, putting pressure on the other toes of the foot.

POINTERS ON PAIN

You can also have a bunion at the base of your little toe. This bunion is called a bunionette.

In addition to being unattractive, bunions cause pain, and you may find walking uncomfortable. The skin can thicken at the base of the big toe and the entire area may become inflamed. A callous can develop at the point where the big toe rubs against the second toe.

The pressure exerted by the big toe against the rest of the toes can cause the rest of the toenails on the affected foot to grow into the sides of the nail bed. These toes can also become deformed and be forced into a clawlike position, a condition referred to as hammertoe.

The primary cause of bunions is ill-fitting shoes, along with arthritis, congenital foot deformity, and trauma. Diagnosis of bunions is fairly straightforward. An x-ray can give further information as to the cause; for example, rheumatoid arthritis as opposed to injury.

Treatment involves changing to better-fitting shoes, orthotics, and NSAIDs, such as naproxen or ibuprofen. Surgery may be necessary if the problem is severe.

Ingrown Toenails

This is a common, painful problem. Pressure, usually on the big toe, forces the edges of the toenail to grow into the skin. The two primary causes of ingrown toenails are ill-fitting shoes with pointy toes and incorrect nail trimming. Other causes include injury and congenital abnormalities of the toe.

The skin around the toenail becomes inflamed and sensitive to any kind of pressure. Diagnosis is fairly straightforward based upon appearance and symptoms. If you are a diabetic, an ingrown toenail is a potentially serious foot problem and should be seen by your doctor.

Treatment involves removing the source of the irritation by changing to properly fitting shoes and trimming the toenail straight across. Nails shouldn't be trimmed so closely that the edges have the opportunity to become ingrown.

Antibiotic ointments are helpful for treating infected ingrown toenails. Soaking the foot in warm water can help relieve symptoms of inflammation. In some cases, surgically removing the embedded portion of the nail may be necessary.

Prevention

Many knee and ankle injuries are the result of overuse during exercise or physical activity. Scaling back on the intensity of workouts and proper warm-ups and cool-downs can go a long way toward preventing these types of injuries. For many foot problems, the repeated advice throughout this chapter has been to wear shoes that fit properly and that are designed for the specific activity for which you'll be using them.

Maintaining a proper weight will take strain off knees and ankles, relieve your pain, and even help prevent osteoarthritis.

You should never have to "break in" your shoes. They should fit properly from the outset and not cause you discomfort. This is the simplest and most economical means of preventing many foot problems and also the principal means of treating existing ones.

If you are a diabetic, be vigilant in checking your feet and skin between the toes for sores, as these can often be overlooked. Because diabetes causes decreased sensation, improper footwear can cause mild open lesions which need to be taken care of immediately. Often family members can help with weekly foot checks.

Treatment

Rest is the first line of treatment for much knee, shin, and foot pain, since many problems here are a result of overuse or misuse. Keeping your leg elevated will help reduce swelling. NSAIDs, such as naproxen or ibuprofen, will also work to control swelling, inflammation, and pain.

Your physician may refer you to a physical therapist to help you work on proper stretching exercises. You may also wish to consult a personal fitness trainer if you need to develop a sensible exercise regimen tailored to your needs.

Surgery is generally considered to be the last option, after more conservative measures have been tried. For a complete discussion of these surgeries, see Chapter 9.

The Least You Need to Know

- Many leg injuries, including shin splints, are caused by overuse. Slow down, scale back, and you'll prevent many of them.
- Falls are the principal cause of ankle injuries. Wearing appropriate footwear for the activity can give more support to this vulnerable joint.
- Weekly foot checks can help diabetics prevent serious foot problems.
- Changing to sensible footwear can both prevent and heal knee and foot problems.
- P.R.I.C.E. (Protection, Rest, Ice, Compression, and Elevation) is your first line of defense in recuperating from knee, shin, ankle, and foot injuries.

Skin Pain

In This Chapter

- Dealing with burns
- Cuts and scrapes
- Skin infections
- Viral infections

Your skin is the largest organ in your body, and it's a prime candidate for injury and infection. In addition, nerve endings in your skin can send pain signals to your brain. Certain medical conditions can cause skin pain, and some of these can be stubborn to treat. In this chapter, you'll learn how to get relief and soothe your painful skin.

When to See the Doctor

Immediate medical attention is required in the case of chemical burns or any burns affecting the eyes. Burns to the face or neck may cause swelling that can obstruct breathing. Seek immediate medical care.

In the case of cuts, if you can't get the bleeding to stop within 10 minutes by placing pressure on it or if the blood is spurting and bright red in color, consider it an emergency situation and seek medical attention. Also, if you are on a blood thinner, you may want to seek medical attention sooner if the bleeding doesn't stop quickly. Blood thinners interfere with the clotting (coagulation) process.

Other situations that require medical attention include any wound that needs suturing. If you can see bone, ligaments, fat, or other tissue through the cut, you'll need to be treated by a physician. If not attended to quickly, this type of injury could lead to a painful infection. Puncture wounds also should be seen by a physician.

If any foreign material, such as dirt, gravel, glass, or other substance, has entered the wound and you can't clean it out thoroughly, a physician can clean it for you.

Diagnosis

Your skin is strong and resilient. It's your body's protective covering, holding all your internal organs snugly in place and keeping harmful viruses and other pathogens out. In addition, your skin helps regulate body temperature. When your skin is damaged, either as the result of injury or infection, it can't operate efficiently, and the pain you feel is an indicator that it needs some help.

Sources of Skin Pain

Your skin is composed of three layers. The outer layer is called the epidermis and contains no blood vessels. It helps to guard against infection and helps maintain body temperature. The middle layer is the dermis, where nerves and blood vessels are located. It's also where your hair follicles and sweat glands reside. This layer helps provide sensations of heat and touch. The third layer is called the hypodermis. It's home to bigger blood vessels and nerves. One of its functions is regulating your body's temperature. It also attaches the skin to the underlying bone and muscle.

As tough as your skin is, it's still vulnerable. Common painful skin injuries include cuts, scrapes, puncture wounds, and burns. These wounds may be superficial or extend deep into the tissues.

Generally, the location of the injury, the amount of surface area involved, and the depth of the injury determine how serious it is.

Shingles

The nerve pain associated with shingles is excruciating. If you had chickenpox as a child, you can develop shingles as an adult. The chickenpox virus (varicella-zoster, or VZV, which is in the herpes family of viruses) never leaves your body, even though you recover from the disease. The virus rests dormant in your central nervous system (CNS). For reasons not fully understood, in later life, this virus comes back with a vengeance as shingles. Early treatment can shorten the duration and intensity of the pain associated with shingles.

Shingles is extremely painful and usually erupts as a burning band of blisters on one side of your body. Most often these blisters can extend from the middle of your back and around one side of your body to a point near your breastbone. Shingles can also affect other nerves around the body and thus other skin areas such as the face, low back, and groin. Sometimes the blisters occur on the face or neck or around one eye. People who get shingles typically say that the worst pain is after the blisters heal. The nerve pain in shingles is known to be the most severe of all nerve pain problems in medicine.

Risk factors for shingles include having had chickenpox as a child, having a suppressed immune system, and being an adult over the age of 50. Your risk increases with age.

Shingles is diagnosed based on an evaluation of your symptoms and a physical examination. Shingles, like chickenpox, is a contagious disease, so be careful not to infect others. Once the blisters have scabbed and crusted over, the contagious period has passed. Pregnant women and infants should not come in contact with someone who has shingles.

Interestingly, anyone who becomes infected as a result of coming in direct contact with the blisters of shingles and who hasn't been vaccinated against chickenpox may contract chickenpox. If you have already had chickenpox, you won't get it again by being around someone with shingles, nor will you get shingles.

There is no way to determine whether an attack of shingles will be mild or severe, but complications can occur in either case. These can include infection, neurological problems, and a painful skin condition called postherpetic neuralgia.

STABS AND JABS

An outbreak of shingles around your eye can cause an eye infection. It's especially important to seek early medical attention to prevent permanent damage to your vision.

Neurological complications can be troublesome and serious. These can include balance problems, hearing difficulties, encephalitis (inflammation of the brain), or facial paralysis. Seeking treatment early on in the course of shingles can help prevent these complications.

Shingles is treated with antiviral medications, including Famciclovir (Famvir), Acyclovir (Zovirax), or Valacyclovir (Valtrex). These medications should be started during the earliest stages of the disease, preferably within 72 hours.

The most common complication of shingles is postherpetic neuralgia. Postherpetic neuralgia refers to the nerve pain that persists more than a month after shingles has occurred. This pain may continue long after the blisters and rash have healed.

People who have suffered from postherpetic neuralgia often describe it as a sharp burning and stabbing pain worse than anything else they have felt. Treatment options include cool compresses or soaking in cool water. Over-the-counter pain medications, along with an oral antihistamine (such as Benadryl) and calamine lotion, or a numbing topical cream or ointment to relieve the itch, can be helpful.

If over-the-counter pain medications don't provide the necessary relief, prescription pain relievers, along with antidepressant or anticonvulsant medications, are available. These work by calming the nerve endings and interrupting the pain cycle.

Today, a vaccine (varicella vaccine) is given to children to protect them against chickenpox. This vaccine is also recommended for adults who have not had chickenpox as children.

If you've had chickenpox, the shingles vaccine (varicella-zoster vaccine), which is a live vaccine, is the recommended option for adults over 60.

POINTERS ON PAIN

No vaccine can guarantee 100 percent immunity. However, even if it doesn't prevent the disease, it can shorten its course, decrease the severity of your symptoms, and lessen your chances of developing complications.

You should not get the shingles vaccination if you have any autoimmune disease, have HIV/AIDS, have cancer, or are on long-term corticosteroids. If you are undergoing chemotherapy or radiation treatment or have had lymphatic or bone marrow cancer, you are not a candidate for the shingles vaccination. Before receiving the vaccination, tell your doctor if you have any known allergies.

Burns

Burns are common, painful skin injuries. Many burns are minor, such as the burn you receive when you brush against a hot iron, sip a drink that's too hot, get a spatter of grease on your hand while cooking, or spend too much time in the sun without sunscreen. It's instant pain, and that pain is your body's message to stop whatever you're doing that's causing the problem.

With first-degree burns, the damage is confined to the outer skin layer. The skin becomes inflamed, hurts to touch, and may swell slightly. Your skin may feel tight and hot, and there's a searing quality to the acute pain.

First-degree burns, although painful, will generally heal on their own, if they are kept clean and protected. For a first-degree burn or a small second-degree burn, wash the area gently using lukewarm water and then apply a topical antibiotic ointment. If the area is likely to rub against clothing, you can cover it with a loose, sterile dressing.

POINTERS ON PAIN

Burns are ranked as first, second, third, fourth, and fifth degree based on their depth. Regardless of the degree, all burns are breaks in the skin and present the possibility of infection.

Second-degree burns are more serious because they go deeper. They have the characteristics of first-degree burns, but they also raise blisters on the skin. The pain of a second-degree burn is more severe and intense than that of a first-degree burn. The nerves may throb, and the searing pain can be intense. The skin feels hot and tight and the blisters may weep if punctured. If this happens, the skin becomes hypersensitive to touch and even air can be painful. A second-degree burn should be evaluated by your physician.

Third-degree burns cause significant damage. They penetrate through the final layer of skin, damage the blood vessels and nerves in the hypodermis, and kill all three layers of skin tissue, which then takes on a white, leatherlike appearance. Ironically, because the area is dead, third-degree burns may not be especially painful, although the skin around these burns may be severely painful. Recovery from third-degree burns can be long and arduous. In severe cases, to avoid shock, burn patients are placed in a medically induced coma to help get through the period of intense pain that comes with treatment and recovery.

Damage caused by burns can continue over a period of some time, and the degree of the burn may change as a result. If a first-degree burn later develops blisters, it has become a second-degree burn. Second-degree burns can also become third-degree burns.

STABS AND JABS

Contrary to what you may have been taught as a child, don't put butter on a burn. It puts up a barrier that repels water and can promote infection by trapping pathogens on the skin.

Second- and third-degree burns are generally treated differently from first-degree burns and require immediate medical attention.

Keep jewelry out of the burn area. Swelling is part of the body's inflammatory response, and if you've burned a finger and keep your ring on, you may find it impossible to get off. You also run the risk of cutting off your circulation.

Chemical burns require immediate medical attention. In the case of chemical burns, first identify the chemical involved and then either call your hospital or the U.S. National Poison Hotline for emergency assistance. You can reach the hotline at 1-800-222-1222.

Electrical burns can damage nerves and muscles, and the damage may not show up immediately. Serious electrical burns should be evaluated by a physician.

Scalding

Scalding accounts for a considerable number of burns incurred in the kitchen. Boiling water, hot coffee or tea, or hot grease can cause serious burns. A scald is a burn and its treatment depends on the degree of the burn.

For a simple scald, run cool (not cold) water over the burn. Then treat as a regular first-degree burn (see the preceding section). However, if blistering occurs, seek medical treatment.

Sunburn

Your body has a protective substance, called melanin, that helps keep the sun's ultraviolet rays from damaging your skin. Excessive sun exposure, however, can surpass the capability of melanin to protect you. Generally, the darker your skin, the longer it takes for you to get a sunburn, but the cumulative effects of sun exposure extend far beyond sunburn. Risks of skin cancer, including melanoma, increase with the amount of time you spend in the sun.

Preventing sunburn is much more desirable than treating it. Use sunblock with a high SPF (sun protection factor) if you're going to be venturing outdoors—even on a cloudy day! Ultraviolet rays are still out there, even if you can't see the sun.

POINTERS ON PAIN

Ultraviolet rays can penetrate thin clothing, so be sure to cover up adequately when in the sun. New lines of clothing with sun-protective capabilities are now being produced and provide excellent protection from UV rays.

After you've noticed that your skin is red and hot, the first step is to get yourself out of the sun as quickly as possible. Cool, damp compresses applied to the sunburned area can relieve some of the discomfort, and a cool shower or bath may also provide help.

If blisters form, keep the skin dry and protected by applying a light dressing. An application of lotion or cream may soothe skin that isn't blistered, but avoid any petroleum-based ointments (such as petroleum jelly), along with lidocaine or benzocaine. These products seal in the heat—something you don't want to do.

Cuts

Just like burns, cuts are breaks in the skin, and their seriousness depends upon how deep they are, how long they are, what caused them, and their location. Most of the time cuts are a minor problem, as when snipping yourself while cutting with scissors or slicing an onion. Washing the wound with soap and water and applying a dressing to help keep it clean while healing is usually all that's necessary.

Deep or gaping cuts that slice through the epidermis and the other two skin layers may damage nerves and blood vessels; if the cut goes deeper, tendons and muscles may also be involved. These types of cuts should be evaluated by a physician.

Location is another important factor to consider. If the cut is situated at a joint (the knee, wrist, elbow, or ankle, for instance), each time you flex or move that joint you're going to disrupt the healing process. Sutures may be necessary to keep the edges of the cut together while they heal.

 STABS AND JABS

A bite, being a puncture wound, counts as a cut. Whether from an animal or a human, a bite can be a source of infection and requires medical attention.

Common sense needs to be your guide. If you've sliced off a finger tip, applying a dressing and "toughing it out" isn't a smart thing to do. In the same vein, regardless of what you've seen on television and in the movies, applying a tourniquet to stop bleeding requires specialized knowledge to prevent causing more damage than help. Applying pressure to the cut is the better method. Place a clean cloth over the cut and press firmly until the bleeding has stopped.

If the bleeding has not stopped within 5 to 10 minutes, seek medical assistance. Also seek medical attention for a "spurting" type of bleeding, which is an indication that an artery has been severed.

> **POINTERS ON PAIN**
>
> Do you have a first-aid kit handy? You should have one at home, in your car, and in any recreational vehicles you use. The time to get one is before you need it. If you need a refresher first-aid course, call your local chapter of the American Red Cross.

For less serious cuts, after you've gotten the bleeding stopped, it's time for a visual examination of the wound. Rinse the cut with lukewarm water and check for any foreign material, such as dirt, gravel, glass, or other matter. Use tweezers to remove foreign matter.

Next, rinse the wound again with lukewarm water and finish with an antiseptic wipe. Sterile gauze is the best material for cleaning the wound. Cleaning the cut may start it bleeding again, so apply pressure once again to stop the bleeding.

If foreign material is deeply embedded in the cut and you're not able to get it all out, seek medical attention to prevent infection.

> **STABS AND JABS**
>
> Scrapes are abrasions. They don't slice through the skin, but they do rough it up. Clean a scrape with lukewarm water and an antiseptic wipe. Scrapes can "weep" as they heal. Keep them clean and use a topical antibiotic to promote faster healing.

Applying an antibiotic ointment to the cut can help prevent infection and can speed healing by as much as five days. Then comes the closure. Closing a minor cut has gotten much easier with the advent of skin strips. These are sticky pieces of tape that can be directly applied to the skin and work very well if the cut is in an area that doesn't get much movement. Skin glue is another option for these types of cuts. Steri-strips or butterfly strips are often used for minor cuts on the face.

For cuts that are long or deep and that are situated above joints, sutures are the standard means of closure.

Sometimes, in spite of your best efforts, the wound can become infected. If you notice that the skin around the cut has become warm and red or see any pus seeping from it, seek medical attention. The most common causes of secondary infection are staph and strep, which require treatment with either prescription or over-the-counter antibiotics.

A thin, red line leading away from a wound generally is an indicator of a skin infection and can be a sign that bacteria have entered the lymph system. In addition to the pain from the wound, you may experience fever and other symptoms of infection. This situation requires medical attention and antibiotics.

Cellulitis

Cellulitis is the medical term for a skin infection that generally occurs after an abrasion, deep cut, or puncture wound. Bacteria enter the body through the open wound, and the skin becomes inflamed. Staph and strep infections are the usual types of bacteria involved. In addition to inflammation, symptoms also include a low-grade fever. Treatment is with antibiotics.

Dermatitis (Eczema)

The terms dermatitis and eczema are often used interchangeably. While eczema is usually associated with infants, this burning, itching condition can occur in adults.

There are several different types of dermatitis. Symptoms include dry, itchy skin; redness; and a burning sensation. The areas most commonly affected include the face, neck, and ankles and the inside of the knees and elbows. With continued scratching, the skin can thicken and become leathery.

Diagnosis is made based upon an evaluation of symptoms and a physical examination. A *skin biopsy* may also be taken to rule out other skin conditions as the source of the pain and itching.

DEFINITION

A **skin biopsy** is a procedure in which a small sample of skin tissue is removed and sent to a lab for analysis.

Treatment involves using lotions and ointments with a low water and high oil content, along with recommendations to shower or bathe less frequently, as these good hygiene habits strip the skin of essential protective oils. It's ironic, but water dries out your skin and can make eczema worse.

When you do shower or bathe, use warm water instead of hot and limit your time in the water. Dry off gently, patting your skin dry instead of rubbing with a towel, and complete your toilette with an application of lotion.

The primary goal of treatment is to get you to stop scratching. Corticosteroid ointments may be prescribed to counteract the skin's inflammatory response along with antihistamines to relieve itching. Benadryl has been shown to be helpful in this regard. An oral corticosteroid or cyclosporine, an immunosuppressant, may be prescribed if the outbreak is severe. Light therapy, also called phototherapy, has been shown to be helpful in relieving symptoms.

> **SPEAKING OF PAIN**
>
> There seems to be a genetic component for eczema, and it's more common in adults with other allergies, including asthma.

Psoriasis

There are many different forms of psoriasis, but the most common one is plaque psoriasis. Other types are classified as pustular, nonpustular, and other (which includes drug-induced psoriasis). The classic symptoms of plaque psoriasis include scaly, thick, red patches. The scales take on a silver or white color as the cells die and the skin continues to build up underneath. These scales can develop anywhere on the body. They often are symmetrical, which means the pattern of distribution is even across both sides of your body. Psoriasis is not contagious.

Psoriasis is not well understood. For some reason, something triggers the immune system to speed up the production of skin cells, and these cells build up into thickened layers. In individuals without psoriasis, a skin cell is born, matures, dies, and sloughs away in about a month's time. In individuals with psoriasis, this whole process takes place in just a few days, except for the shedding part. These skin cells hang on and stack up.

Risk factors for developing psoriasis are far-ranging and can include prior skin injury, stress, allergies, and a strep infection. In addition, certain medications can trigger an outbreak of psoriasis. These include the following:

- Antimalarial medications—Used in treating rheumatoid arthritis, lupus, and other autoimmune disorders in addition to malaria. These medications include Plaquenil, chloroquine, hydroxychloroquine, and Quinacrine.

- Lithium—Used in treating bipolar depression and other psychiatric conditions.

- Inderal—Used to treat high blood pressure.

- Indomethacin—A nonsteroidal anti-inflammatory drug (NSAID) used to treat arthritis.

- Quinidine—Used to treat heart disease.

SPEAKING OF PAIN

According to the National Institutes of Health, psoriasis affects as many as 7.5 million Americans.

Certain environmental allergens, such as cold weather, may also trigger an attack of psoriasis. Obesity has been associated with certain types of psoriasis. Smoking has also been implicated as a trigger, along with heavy consumption of alcohol.

Diagnosis is made based upon an evaluation of symptoms and a physical examination. You may be referred to a *dermatologist* for evaluation and treatment.

DEFINITION

A **dermatologist** is a physician specializing in treating diseases of the skin.

Treatment is focused on breaking the accelerated production of skin cells, controlling the itch, and returning the skin to a normal appearance. Antihistamines, corticosteroids, topical preparations containing capsaicin, antidepressants, and topical anesthetics can be helpful.

Corticosteroids delivered in lotion form are extremely helpful in treating psoriasis. They work by slowing down skin cell production, reducing inflammation, and relieving itching. Other treatments include the following:

- Anthralin
- Vitamin D
- Tazarotene (Tazorac, Avage)
- Coal tar
- Salicylic acid

- Methotrexate
- Cyclosporine
- Hydroxyurea
- Light therapy

A class of drugs called the biologics has shown promise in treating psoriasis by interfering with certain immune cell functions. These medications are generally administered intravenously or by injection. Commonly prescribed biologics include alefacept (Amevive), infliximab (Remicade), and etanercept (Enbrel).

Psoriasis cannot be cured, but its symptoms can be managed. Your best resource for information on current research, treatments, and coping suggestions is the National Psoriasis Foundation (www.psoriasis.org).

Prevention

Falls, accidents, and burns are the primary causes of skin pain. Protecting your skin from injury is the first line of defense. Cover up when you're in the sunshine and apply sunblock to protect against sunburn. If you're a sports enthusiast, wear the proper protective gear to help prevent skin injuries.

Treatment

Prompt treatment of injuries can help relieve skin pain. If you're not up on your first aid, the time to take a refresher course is before you need it. Check with your local chapter of the American Red Cross for a schedule of classes. Their website is www.redcross.org.

Keep current on your medications if your skin pain is the result of a medical condition, and check with your doctor if your medications aren't doing the job.

The Least You Need to Know

- Burns of any type that involve the eyes require immediate medical attention.
- Cellulitis is a skin infection caused by the staph or strep bacteria. It requires treatment with antibiotics.
- Vaccination can help protect against the shingles virus.
- Corticosteroids and a class of medications called the biologics are helpful in treating the symptoms of psoriasis.

Abdominal Pain

In This Chapter

- Avoiding hernias
- Ulcers and infection
- When bleeding is a concern
- STDs and pain

Your abdomen is home not only to nerves, bones, muscles, tendons, and ligaments, but also to many vital internal organs. Here, infection as well as malfunction can cause you pain; a stomachache can be a symptom of something much more serious than overeating. In this chapter, we'll take an in-depth look at what can cause pain in your tummy and how to go about getting relief.

When to See the Doctor

Symptoms that require immediate medical attention include sharp abdominal pain that comes on suddenly or abdominal pain accompanied by pain in your chest, shoulder, or neck. If there is blood in your stool or if you are vomiting blood, consider it an emergency situation. If your abdomen is tight, bloated, and hurts when you touch it, you should also seek immediate medical care.

Call your doctor if you have abdominal pain and any of these additional symptoms:

- Fever
- No appetite
- Diarrhea

- Unplanned weight loss

- Frequent urination or burning with urination

Use common sense. If your abdomen is uncomfortable for more than a few days and you haven't been overindulging in food or drink, check with your doctor.

 STABS AND JABS

If you are pregnant or could be pregnant, any abdominal pain should be evaluated by your physician.

Diagnosis

Diagnosing the source of abdominal pain can be a challenging process both for the patient and the physician. The starting point is an evaluation of symptoms, followed by a review of your medical history and a physical examination. To find out why it hurts, your physician must first find out where it hurts and when it hurts. She does this by asking some probing questions.

Where Does It Hurt?

Even allowing for some small individual variations, most people's anatomical layout follows the same pattern. Your abdomen is considered to begin just below your ribs and end just above your pubic bone. It extends across the front of your body to your sides.

Your abdomen is a cavity; in fact, it's referred to as the abdominal cavity, because it's a hollow space that holds several essential internal organs. Each of these organs, such as your gallbladder or pancreas, for example, occupies a particular spot within the abdominal cavity.

By pointing to your upper abdomen on the right side, you're telling the doctor that the problem might be your gallbladder. If you point to your upper abdomen and also mention that your back is hurting, this may be a clue that your pancreas is the source of your pain. Again, these are only some of the possibilities. Pain can also refer from one place to another, so this is only one way of thinking about the cause of your abdominal pain.

If you're having trouble pinpointing the exact location, don't hesitate to tell your doctor. Telling your doctor that the pain seems to be coming from different directions or that you simply can't isolate it can be helpful information.

When Does It Hurt?

Sometimes pain comes and goes. This intermittent pain can be frustrating to diagnose. For example, do you feel bloated and experience sharp abdominal pain after eating? The problem might be gas. If you feel pain around the time of your bowel movement, the problem could be constipation.

On the other hand, abdominal pain that doesn't let up in intensity might be caused by anything from a kidney stone to appendicitis.

Pain that gets worse when you move might indicate a strained muscle or a hernia. It can also be an indicator of inflammation somewhere in your abdominal cavity.

Describing the Pain

It's important to be as accurate and as honest as you can in describing what the pain feels like—whether it's a dull ache or a sharp, severe jolt. Everyone's experience with pain is unique, but many medical conditions share some common aspects. The kind of pain you're feeling gives some important clues.

Not every serious abdominal problem is accompanied by serious pain. Sometimes there's little if any pain at all; for example, cancer of the colon in its early stages is painless, while the pain of less serious conditions, such as heartburn, can be excruciating.

It's also important to talk to your doctor about the associated symptoms that you could be having. Some of these symptoms include nausea, fatigue, change in appetite, fever, chills, vomiting, feeling of fullness, changes in bowel habits, or changes in bowel movement color.

POINTERS ON PAIN

Don't be squeamish or reticent when it comes to discussing body functions with your doctor. She's heard it all before.

Next Steps

After a complete physical examination, you may be asked for a urine and/or stool sample, which is then sent to the lab for analysis. Most likely you'll have blood drawn to check your complete blood count (CBC) and some other labs to check your liver functions.

A high white blood cell count can indicate the presence of infection, and if your liver and pancreas enzymes are elevated, this can be a sign of inflammation. Other tests may include x-rays, CT scan, *colonoscopy*, or an upper GI series. If none of these are conclusive, exploratory surgery may be necessary to get to the source of the problem.

> **DEFINITION**
>
> A **colonoscopy** is a procedure in which the physician inserts a flexible tube equipped with a camera into the rectum and up into the colon to look for abnormalities. The pictures are transmitted to a computer screen in real time.

Sources of Abdominal Pain

Your abdomen is host to numerous internal organs, including your stomach, gallbladder, pancreas, intestines, appendix, reproductive organs, liver, spleen, kidneys, adrenal glands, and lymph nodes—all neatly wrapped in muscle and protected by a layer of fat and your skin. Any one of these tenants can have a malfunction, incur an injury or an infection, or be in need of repair. In many cases, the first sign you have of a problem is pain.

Hernia

The muscles that protect the abdomen are strong, but occasionally a tear or a congenital weakness here sets the stage for a hernia, which occurs when that tear or weakness opens up and allows some portion of internal organ (often the intestine) or tissue to protrude through that hole. If large enough, you will see a bulging at the spot. Any type of exertion, such as bending or lifting, puts added strain on the spot and will tend to make the pain worse. This bulging can also occur after any surgery that makes the muscle weak in that area.

STABS AND JABS

When part of the intestine or other tissue from the abdomen gets caught in the hernia, it can have its blood supply interrupted. This serious complication requires surgery immediately to correct the problem before the tissue dies from blood loss.

Most often hernias develop in the groin area of the lower abdomen, an area with less muscle support, although they can occur in several other locations in the abdomen. After a hernia has developed, surgical repair is the only way to correct the problem.

Diagnosis is made based upon an evaluation of symptoms and a physical examination. You may be asked to cough, as coughing often causes the bulge to become larger as more strain is delivered to the affected area.

Hernias may have a genetic component, which means that if other members of your family have had them, you may be more likely to develop one. Men with an enlarged prostate are at increased risk for hernia. If you have a chronic cough, are overweight, suffer from constipation, or if your occupation requires you to perform heavy lifting, you may also be at increased risk.

Prevention is always a good approach when warding off pain. You may not be able to control many risk factors, such as your genetics, but there are some things you can do. You can be sure to include enough fiber in your diet so you don't get constipated. You can also maintain a proper weight. If your job requires you to lift, always wear a hernia support and lift with your legs—not your back.

Treatment for a hernia involves surgery to push the protruding organ or tissue back through the opening and repair the hole. It's important to have this done before complications occur. The success rate for hernia surgery is excellent.

Ulcers

An ulcer is an open sore, and it can develop in any of your body's mucous membranes, such as in your mouth, your stomach, or your duodenum, which is part of your small intestine. The three types of ulcers are gastric (stomach), duodenal, and peptic (ulcers that occur in the lining of the stomach or duodenum). Your body uses naturally occurring acids in these locations to help digest your food. These acids, hydrochloric acid and pepsin, contribute to ulcer growth.

Side effects of over-the-counter and prescription nonsteroidal anti-inflammatory drugs (NSAIDs), such as ibuprofen, naproxen, and aspirin, include stomach irritation and stomach ulcers.

To help prevent the development of peptic ulcers as a complication of NSAID use, ask your doctor about the benefits a proton pump inhibitor (PPI) may give. A PPI is a class of medication that blocks an acid-producing enzyme in the stomach wall. Reducing the amount of acid can help ulcers heal and help prevent formation of new ulcers. The following are commonly prescribed PPIs:

- Prilosec (omeprazole)

- Nexium (esomeprazole)

- Prevacid (lansoprazole)

- Protonix (pantoprazole)

- Aciphex (lansoprazole)

SPEAKING OF PAIN

Although stomach ulcers develop more often in women, duodenal ulcers develop more often in men. Regardless of your sex, you have a 1 in 10 chance of developing an ulcer in your lifetime.

You may have heard that ulcers are a lifestyle affliction, caused by too much stress and worry along with poor dietary choices. Today we know that although these provide optimum growing conditions for ulcers, the main culprit is infection caused by a bacterium called *Heliobacter pylori* or *H. pylori* for short.

After you've got an ulcer, however, certain things, such as alcohol, caffeine, and smoking, can aggravate your symptoms.

Ulcer pain is generally a burning sensation that's located just below the rib cage. Often this burning pain is at its most severe midway between meals, and it tends to come and go. Sometimes this pain is accompanied by belching or nausea.

If you've been experiencing this type of pain, you may have mistaken it for heartburn or simple gas, and if you've been treating it with antacids, you may have gotten some relief. However, ulcers require different treatment to avoid some serious complications. Stomach or duodenal ulcers that have spread to surrounding blood vessels can damage those vessels, resulting in bleeding.

STABS AND JABS

When an ulcer erodes the stomach or intestinal wall, bacteria from these locations can cause infection within the abdominal cavity. This serious infection, called peritonitis, can be fatal. Seek treatment early to help prevent infection.

Diagnostic procedures for ulcers focus on identifying the cause of the ulcer, in addition to determining its location, so an effective treatment protocol can be developed. In addition to an evaluation of symptoms and a physical examination, an upper GI series may be necessary, along with testing tissue samples to determine whether the bacteria *H. pylori* is present. This can be done with a breath test or a blood test.

If *H. pylori* is present, antibiotics are given to kill the bacteria. Other medications include acid blockers to either inhibit or neutralize acids in the stomach or intestine. In some cases, surgery may be necessary to repair an ulcer.

Appendicitis

Your appendix used to be considered a vestigial organ—a remnant that's no longer needed and is just occupying space in your abdomen. New research has disproved that, however, and your appendix may play a significant role in fighting infection.

The appendix is a wormlike pouch attached to the cecum, which is the beginning of the large intestine. Thus the name "vermiform appendix." Your appendix is usually located in the lower right side of your abdomen, although its placement varies from individual to individual.

Appendicitis is an inflammation of the appendix, and the pain associated with this condition generally comes on quickly, is severe, and gets worse. Fever, nausea, vomiting, and swelling in the abdomen are other symptoms. Left untreated, the appendix can rupture, resulting in peritonitis, a life-threatening condition.

SPEAKING OF PAIN

Peritonitis is the most common cause of abdominal emergencies among children and young adults. It is most common in males age 10 to 14 and females between the ages of 15 and 19.

Diagnosis is based upon an evaluation of the symptoms and a physical examination. Blood work may be ordered, with a high white blood cell count indicating the presence of infection or inflammation. Diagnostic imaging tests may be indicated if the symptoms mimic those of another condition, such as inflammatory bowel disease or an intestinal obstruction. Time is of the essence in diagnosing and treating appendicitis.

Treatment involves surgical removal of the appendix followed by a course of antibiotics to treat any infection that may be present.

Gallbladder

The gallbladder rests right under your liver, in the upper right part of your abdomen. Shaped rather like a pear, its job is to store and release the bile produced by your liver. This bile is necessary for your body to digest fat. During the digestive process, the gallbladder releases bile by means of a tube called the common bile duct. This tube is shared by your liver, and your gallbladder and connects them to the small intestine.

A gallbladder attack usually can be traced to something obstructing the passage of the bile through the common bile duct. *Gallstones* are the usual culprits, although tumors in the pancreas or the bile duct can also be the source of the pain. Inflammation of the gallbladder (cholecystitis) is also a possibility.

DEFINITION

A **gallstone** is a solid crystal deposit, usually made up of cholesterol. Gallstones can range from the size of a grain of sand to the size of a golf ball.

Risk factors for developing gallbladder disease include being a woman age 40 and younger, being overweight, having diabetes, and having a diet high in saturated fats and sugars.

Diagnosis is based upon an evaluation of your symptoms, a physical examination, blood work, and one or more diagnostic imaging tests. One of these tests, called the HIDA (Hepatobiliary Iminodiacetic Acid) scan, shows how effectively bile is being moved down the bile duct.

As with other diagnostic imaging procedures that use contrast material or a radioactive tracer to obtain clearer pictures, there are some precautions you should be aware of. You should not have a HIDA scan if you are pregnant or think you may be pregnant. Tell your physician if you are allergic to any contrast materials that may be used. (See Chapter 4 for a complete discussion of imaging tests and precautions.)

Another diagnostic test used for gallbladder disease is an endoscopic ultrasound. The doctor inserts the endoscope (a thin, flexible tube with a tiny camera attached) into your mouth or your rectum and then guides it to the area under study. Pictures are transmitted to a computer, which gives a real-time display of the procedure.

You can do quite a bit to help safeguard against gallbladder disease. Choose a diet high in fiber and include plenty of fresh fruits and vegetables. In addition, other healthy choices include the following:

- Omega-3 fatty acids—found in fatty fish, such as salmon

- Olive or canola oils

- Nuts—including peanuts, walnuts, and almonds

Research has come up with some interesting statistics regarding the effects of alcohol and coffee consumption on the gallbladder. Moderate alcohol consumption, which has been defined as one to two drinks a day, has been linked with a 20 percent reduced risk of gallbladder disease in women. For coffee, it appears that the caffeine plays a role in stimulating gallbladder contractions and lowering the cholesterol content in the bile. For some reason researchers do not yet understand, the caffeine needs to come from coffee to be effective, which means that tea and other caffeinated beverages don't have the same beneficial effect.

Treatment of gallbladder disease may involve endoscopic surgery to remove a gallstone or other obstruction. Ursodiol is a medication used to dissolve gallstones, and a procedure called lithotripsy can be used to pulverize solitary gallstones less than 2 centimeters in diameter.

The gallbladder is not essential to life, so if the gallbladder has become severely inflamed and doesn't respond to treatment, laparoscopic surgery may be performed to remove it, a procedure called cholecystectomy.

Gastrointestinal Bleeding

The gastrointestinal (GI) tract begins near your mouth and terminates at your rectum. Generally the tract is divided into two areas: upper, from your mouth to the upper portion of the small intestine; and lower, from the upper portion of the small intestine to the rectum. Any portion of the GI tract can bleed, and the amounts involved can range from so small that only microscopic analysis can detect it to so great that it poses an imminent threat to life.

STABS AND JABS

Even minuscule bleeding in the GI tract, if prolonged, can result in serious complications, including anemia. Bleeding in the GI tract, however small, should not be ignored.

Severe bleeding from the GI tract may result in vomiting blood or passing blood in the stool, in which case the blood may look like "coffee grounds."

There are many possible reasons for GI tract bleeding, ranging from allergies to hemorrhoids (discussed in the next section) to cancer. If the bleeding is not apparent in your stool, you may not be aware of it until the doctor explains your test results to you. Diagnosis may require blood work, stool analysis, and diagnostic imaging tests, including a colonoscopy.

Treatment of serious gastrointestinal bleeding may include fluids delivered intravenously, blood transfusions, and surgery.

Hemorrhoids

Hemorrhoids often make themselves known when you attempt to have a bowel movement. Pain passing stool and blood in the toilet water are classic symptoms of hemorrhoids, along with severe itching and pain when you sit down.

POINTERS ON PAIN

Constipation can be acutely painful but it's a problem that generally responds well to positive changes in diet.

A hemorrhoid is a swollen vein at the rectum or above it. Bleeding associated with a hemorrhoid is bright red and may be alarming when you see it in the toilet water after a bowel movement. Often, the pain is relieved after the hemorrhoid bleeds, but this relief is only temporary.

For hemorrhoids, stool softeners may be helpful, along with increasing fluid intake and eating a diet high in fiber. If hemorrhoids don't improve, surgical removal may be indicated.

Anal Fissures

Anal fissures are rips in the wall of the rectum. Passing hard stool if you have an anal fissure can be severely painful. You may see bright red blood in your stool with these fissures, although the amounts are small.

For anal fissures, as with hemorrhoids, stool softeners may be helpful, along with increasing fluid intake and eating a diet high in fiber.

Diverticulosis/Diverticulitis

Diverticula is the medical name for pockets that form on the wall of the lower GI tract. If you have these diverticula, you are said to have a medical condition called diverticulosis. As you get older, your chances of having these pockets form increases, and half of us over 60 have diverticulosis. As you strain to have a bowel movement, these diverticuli become inflamed and can bleed. Inflammation of the diverticula is called diverticulitis.

Symptoms can include abdominal pain, usually on the lower left side of the abdomen. Cramps, nausea, fever, chills, and vomiting are additional symptoms, along with a change in bowel habits.

Diagnosis is made based upon symptoms, medical examination, and diagnostic imaging tests such as a colonoscopy, ultrasound, or CT scan.

Switching to a diet high in fiber is an excellent way to begin managing problems in this area.

> **SPEAKING OF PAIN**
>
> How much fiber do you need? The American Dietetic Association recommends 20 to 35 grams of fiber daily.

Increase your consumption of water and other liquids to keep hydrated. Medications include pain relievers and antibiotics.

Gastritis

Gastritis is an inflammation of the wall of the stomach, and it's a common side effect of NSAIDs. Other causes of gastritis include use of alcohol, corticosteroids, trauma, and infection. Symptoms of gastritis include bloating, belching, and nausea, sometimes with vomiting. There can be a burning sensation in the upper abdominal area, along with a feeling of fullness or tightness. In some cases there may be blood in the stool.

Diagnosis is made based on symptoms, medical history, and a physical examination. Blood and stool tests may be ordered. In some cases endoscopy may be necessary to confirm a diagnosis.

Treatment consists of eliminating the causes, such as alcohol or specific foods that trigger the gastritis. Antacids may be helpful in relieving symptoms. If infection, such as *H. pylori*, is the cause, antibiotics may be prescribed.

Pancreatitis

Pancreatitis is inflammation of the pancreas, the gland that's responsible for secreting digestive enzymes that combine with bile produced by the liver to digest your food. When the pancreas becomes inflamed, the enzymes it produces don't go about their normal business, but instead turn on the pancreas and irritate it.

Pancreatitis can be either acute or chronic. Either condition can cause serious harm to the pancreas. Men are more susceptible to both forms.

 SPEAKING OF PAIN

Gallstones are the most common cause of acute pancreatitis.

Symptoms can include fever, nausea and vomiting, an abdomen that's swollen and tender to the touch, and a rapid pulse. This is a serious condition that can lead to shock and death if untreated.

Diagnosis is made based on symptoms, medical history, and a physical examination that may include an abdominal ultrasound or CT scan.

Acute pancreatitis is treated with intravenous (IV) fluids, pain medications, and antibiotics. For chronic pancreatitis, surgery to remove the damaged portion of the pancreas may be required. In severe cases, diabetes may result as a complication of a damaged pancreas.

Irritable Bowel Syndrome

A syndrome is a collection of symptoms with a common cause. Abdominal cramping is a common symptom of irritable bowel syndrome (IBS), along with bloating, gas, and diarrhea or constipation. You may notice some white mucous in your stool and sometimes a sensation that your bowel movement isn't finished.

Diagnosis is generally made after evaluating your symptoms and conducting a physical examination. Your physician may recommend a colonoscopy to rule out other conditions such as cancer. Sometimes, IBS diagnosis can be given because other causes have not been found for your symptoms. If this is the case, making sure you don't have cancer is the first priority before concluding that you have IBS. Remember that although colon cancer is more common among people age 50 and above, persistent abdominal pain should trigger a careful evaluation to rule out cancer. Unfortunately, colon cancer is increasingly common in the adult population in the United States.

Certain foods and drinks can aggravate IBS. These include the following:

- Chocolate
- Greasy foods
- Dairy products
- Caffeine
- Carbonated beverages

IBS is not a life-threatening condition, but it can be painful and make your life uncomfortable. Treatment can include medications, such as antispasmodics that control colon spasms, laxatives or stool softeners, and antidepressants, which can help relieve pain.

Inflammatory Bowel Disease

Ulcerative colitis is one of a group of conditions that fall into the category of inflammatory bowel disease. Crohn's disease is another type of inflammatory bowel disease (IBD). It is thought that IBD is an autoimmune response to bacteria that are normally present in the digestive tract.

Joint pain and cramps in the abdomen are two of the symptoms of IBD, in addition to unexplained weight loss, fatigue, sores on the skin, and rectal bleeding.

Diagnosis is made based upon an evaluation of symptoms, medical examination, blood work, and stool analysis. A colonoscopy is often used to confirm the diagnosis.

Treatment is generally with a class of medications called aminosalicylates (which help to relieve inflammation), immunosuppressants, or corticosteroids. In severe cases, surgery to remove the colon may be necessary.

Pelvic Pain

Your pelvis, located in your lower abdomen, is the place where your reproductive organs are housed. Your pelvic area also includes many of the organs responsible for elimination functions.

Urinary Tract Infections

After you've had one urinary tract infection (UTI), you'll never mistake its symptoms for anything else. You have the sensation that you need to urinate, but little urine is produced. Then the pain comes in an arc, building until it's nearly unbearable, and then subsides. Along with these symptoms, you might have a dull ache in your lower abdomen. When you urinate there is often a burning pain. You may also have pain in your groin and, in severe cases, low back pain as a result of pyelonephritis (infection of the kidney).

Urine contains salts, fluids, and waste products, but it's normally sterile. When bacteria find an entry to the urethra, the tube that carries urine from your bladder to your elimination point, they can quickly multiply and cause an infection. UTIs are more common in women than in men. Most infections here involve the same bacteria—and it's one you're undoubtedly familiar with: *Escherichia coli*, commonly referred to as *E. coli*.

Where does this bacteria come from? In most cases, it comes from your own colon. Women who have a habit of wiping from back to front run the risk of introducing the *E. coli* bacteria into their urinary tract. Therefore, one means of protecting yourself is to get into the habit of wiping from front to back.

Other risk factors for developing a UTI include having a catheter, diabetes, or an autoimmune disease, such as lupus or rheumatoid arthritis.

Following are several types of common UTIs:

- Urethritis—Infection of the urethra

- Cystitis—Infection of the bladder

- Pyelonephritis—Infection of the kidneys

Diagnosis is made based upon evaluation of your symptoms and collection of a urine sample sent for testing. Treatment usually consists of antibacterial medications. It's essential to complete the entire course of antibacterial treatment to prevent a recurrence of your symptoms.

POINTERS ON PAIN

If you are pregnant and develop a UTI, get prompt treatment to avoid the risk of premature labor.

In men, UTIs are frequently due to an obstruction in the urinary tract or an enlarged prostate. Treatment in men can be lengthier and is aimed at preventing inflammation of the prostate.

Interstitial Cystitis

This is the term for a medical condition in which you experience uncomfortable sensations in your bladder and the area around your bladder in the pelvis. These sensations can range from feelings of mild pressure to severe pain. Accompanying these sensations is the feeling that you need to urinate frequently. Interstitial cystitis (IC) is far more common in women than in men. For some women, these symptoms intensify during the menstrual period and during sexual intercourse.

IC may be related to other medical conditions, such as fibromyalgia or IBS, and genetics may play a role in its development, as it tends to run in families.

Diagnosis is made based upon symptoms, a medical examination, urinalysis, and in some cases, a biopsy to rule out other conditions as the source of the problem.

IC does not follow a predictable pattern, and treatment can be difficult. Relieving pain is the primary goal of treatment. Aspirin and NSAIDs can be helpful. Antidepressant medications also may help in relieving symptoms.

Sexually Transmitted Diseases

Pain associated with sexually transmitted diseases varies in location and intensity. It may be felt in the abdomen or as burning during urination. It may show up as sores on your skin or on your genitals. Even if your symptoms are not too troublesome, it's important to remember that a sexually transmitted disease (STD) doesn't cure itself. Unless you get treatment, it's there to stay. Over time an STD can cause serious complications, including sterility, pain, joint and heart damage, and death.

Diagnosis is made based upon physical symptoms, physical examination, and blood work. Some STDs, such as HIV/AIDS, have no cure, but symptoms can be managed and life expectancy extended. Some STDs respond well to medications, although a disturbing trend is emerging concerning medication-resistant strains.

Regardless of what type of STD you are dealing with, your sexual partner (or partners) will also need to be treated.

Prevention

For many abdominal pain issues, a change to a healthier diet will reap substantial benefits. Regular, moderate exercise will bolster your immune system and increase your stamina.

Practicing safer sex will decrease your chances of contracting an STD and having to deal with the pain and potentially life-threatening consequences of these spoilers.

Treatment

Because of the number of internal organs housed in your abdomen, treatment will be determined by the nature of the problem you're experiencing. For some conditions that cannot be diagnosed with a physical examination, blood work, or diagnostic imaging, exploratory endoscopic surgery may be necessary.

The Least You Need to Know

- The severity of abdominal pain is not an accurate indicator of the seriousness of the problem.
- Many common urinary tract infections can be prevented by practicing good bathroom hygiene.

- Increasing the amount of fiber in your diet can help prevent several types of medical conditions that cause abdominal pain.

- Many cases of abdominal pain resulting from infection by a sexually transmitted disease can be prevented by practicing safer sex.

Pain Specific to Women

Chapter 18

In This Chapter

- The role of hormones
- Sources of infections
- When sex hurts
- Pregnancy problems

With the onset of puberty, a woman's body undergoes numerous changes, both internal and external. It is now understood that hormonal changes, physical development, and genetics play a key role in pain syndromes and pain conditions in women. These pain states can occur on a monthly basis or throughout the course of a nine-month pregnancy and sporadically in between. In this chapter, we'll examine the types of pain unique to the female experience and look at ways of getting relief.

When to See the Doctor

Women are no strangers to pain. The monthly cramps that accompany the menses and the pains of childbirth are facts of the female life. However, when monthly pain increases beyond the level you are able to cope with and becomes the focus of your thoughts, or when pain interferes with your ability to go about your life's activities, it's time to check in with your physician.

Diagnosis

Your annual pelvic examination is a key instrument in detecting problems with your reproductive organs. A pelvic exam can detect anything from early pregnancy to abnormalities in your uterus. In addition, sexually active women should have a pap smear done at the time of the annual exam and be vaccinated against the human papilloma virus (HPV).

STABS AND JABS

The similarity of names may cause some confusion. The pap smear is named for Dr. Georgios Papanikolaou, who developed the procedure. A papilloma is a tumor. There is no connection between the two terms.

Infections

Infections involving the female reproductive system run the gamut from an overproduction of naturally occurring bacteria to sexually transmitted diseases. Symptoms alone can't distinguish between these conditions, so it's important to check in with your doctor if you notice anything out of the ordinary.

Vaginitis

Vaginitis is the term used to refer to inflammation or infection of the vagina. Symptoms of vaginitis include burning, itching, and irritation, and, with some kinds of vaginitis, vaginal discharge.

Diagnosis is made based upon evaluation of symptoms, a gynecologic examination, and culture of the vaginal discharge to determine the source of the problem.

Yeast infections are an uncomfortable and common form of vaginitis. The intense itching and burning stem from an overgrowth of candida, which is found normally in the vagina. Other symptoms of candida infection include an odorless thick and white vaginal discharge that looks like cottage cheese. The tissues of the vagina and vulva redden, and the itch can be excruciating.

Treatment for yeast infection is with suppositories or creams inserted by means of an applicator into the vagina. These preparations are available over the counter. Different brands and different treatment schedules are available, ranging from one day to one week. Ask your physician or pharmacist which is your best choice.

POINTERS ON PAIN

Bacteria and yeasts can multiply in damp, warm environments. If you're susceptible to vaginitis, wear cotton underwear and avoid tight-fitting pants.

After you've had one yeast infection, you're not likely to mistake its symptoms should you get another one. Before treating yourself the first time, however, have your physician determine what kind of vaginitis you have, as treatments differ.

Another common form of vaginitis, bacterial vaginitis, is caused by an overgrowth of bacteria that are normally present in the vagina. A characteristic symptom of bacterial vaginitis is a thin whitish discharge with a fishy odor. Treatment for bacterial vaginitis is with antibiotics that must be obtained by prescription.

Vaginitis can also result from an allergic reaction to various irritants, such as detergents, soaps, and fabric softeners. Spermicides, along with vaginal douches and sprays, can also irritate the delicate tissue in this area, causing intense itching, redness, and discharge.

Discovering the triggers from this noninfectious form of vaginitis can take some detective work. If you've recently changed soaps, detergents, or fabric softeners, try switching back to your former brand and see whether the symptoms improve. Your physician can prescribe topical medication to relieve your symptoms.

POINTERS ON PAIN

Contrary to what advertising tells you, the vagina is self-cleaning. Douching and vaginal sprays are a waste of your money and can irritate sensitive tissues. Odor is a symptom of infection. Your physician is the one to determine the cause of this and prescribe treatment.

One form of vaginitis, trichomoniasis, is sexually transmitted, and is caused by a single-celled parasite. Symptoms include intense burning, itching, soreness in the vaginal area, and burning with urination. Some women do not have any symptoms, however.

Because trichomoniasis is a sexually transmitted disease (STD), both you and your partner(s) must be treated. Until you have been cured, you can transmit this infection if you engage in sexual intercourse.

Treatment requires an antibiotic, either tinidazole or metronidazole.

Pelvic Inflammatory Disease

Pelvic inflammatory disease (PID) refers to a bacterial infection located within a woman's reproductive tract. During sexual intercourse, bacteria can enter the vagina, and from there they can migrate to the internal sex organs.

PID is often the result of an STD such as gonorrhea or chlamydia. PID affects more than one million women each year in the United States and is a prime cause of infertility. It can also cause ectopic pregnancy and chronic pain. Risk factors for PID include having had a previous episode of PID, douching, having multiple sexual partners, and having a partner who has or has had multiple partners.

Sometimes there are no symptoms with PID, but pain can occur in the lower abdomen, with urination, and with sexual intercourse.

Diagnosis is made based upon symptoms when present, a pelvic examination, tissue cultures, and diagnostic imaging such as ultrasound. Treatment is with antibiotics. Prevention includes safer sex practices, which can reduce the risk of contracting an STD.

Painful Intercourse

It wasn't all that long ago that a woman would have been told "It's all in your head" or "You're frigid." Thankfully, medical science has proven that sex can indeed hurt sometimes, and it's got nothing to do with your self-esteem as a woman or your inability to embrace your sexual side.

The term for painful intercourse is dyspareunia, and it can occur before penetration, during intercourse, or in the aftermath. There are specific causes and treatments for dyspareunia, and it's important to learn what these are. Left untreated, the emotional fallout can cause serious problems in your relationships and also with your self-esteem.

> **SPEAKING OF PAIN**
>
> It's estimated that nearly 60 percent of women experience pain during sexual intercourse at some time.

Probably the principal cause of pain during intercourse is inadequate lubrication. During intercourse, the vagina secretes fluids that protect the sensitive tissues and allow the penis to move freely without irritating them. These fluids are released during foreplay, as the body's way of preparing for penetration.

If foreplay either doesn't last long enough or isn't effective in stimulating the production of these fluids, penetration is going to hurt. Fluctuations in estrogen levels can be responsible, especially after childbirth or while you're nursing an infant. The problem can become chronic after menopause.

Certain medications can decrease your libido, which can lead to less lubrication and result in painful intercourse. These medications include antidepressants, blood pressure medication, some antihistamines, and those containing narcotics.

Any trauma to your pelvic area, surgery, infection, or skin condition that's causing irritation can also interrupt the smooth flow of your sex life.

> **POINTERS ON PAIN**
>
> Vaginismus are involuntary muscle spasms in the wall of the vagina. They can make attempts at penetration painful.

Sometimes the pain isn't at the point of entry but rather is felt deep inside. Infection in the cervix, fallopian tubes, uterus, or a urinary tract infection may be responsible for this pain and is a signal to get yourself checked out by your physician. Other causes of deep pain include the following:

- Hemorrhoids
- Pelvic inflammatory disease
- Endometriosis
- Uterine problems, such as prolapse, "tipped" uterus, or fibroids
- Ovarian cysts

If you're undergoing chemotherapy or radiation, you may also experience deep pain.

Finally, there is the emotional component of sex. The most important sexual organ in the human body is the brain. How you feel about sex and your partner obviously play a big role in how your body responds during sex.

It's not just sexual feelings that matter, however. If you're worried about your job, if the bills are piling up, if you're having problems with your kids, if you've got health concerns—the list of stressors in life seems to be endless. Sometimes, it's just not possible to turn these concerns off when you settle down for some R&R.

If stress is the cause of the difficulties, you may need more time in intimacy with less concern about performance. Not every sexual episode needs to end in intercourse.

Emotional needs are different from sexual ones, and when the former are addressed, you'll probably find the quality of sex gets better.

Diagnosis of dyspareunia is usually made after discussing your concerns with your doctor, who then will do a thorough physical examination, including a pelvic exam. Sometimes the pelvic portion of the exam is painful. If it hurts, say so. Tell the doctor what you're feeling and how and where it hurts. This can be invaluable diagnostic information.

Diagnostic imaging tests, such as a pelvic ultrasound, may also be indicated to see if any abnormalities in the pelvis are the source of your pain. Treating any infection present is the first step toward relieving your pain.

Treatment options are varied and wide-ranging. First of all, try a lubricant to make penetration easier. K-Y jelly or Astroglide are available over the counter. Both are water-based lubricants.

STABS AND JABS

Petroleum jelly (Vaseline) can cause condoms to break down. It may also contribute to vaginitis, so use a water-based lubricant instead.

Your physician may recommend you practice your Kegels—the exercises that help you strengthen the muscles in the vaginal area. These are the muscles you use when you stop the flow of urine. The stronger they get, the more control you'll have.

These exercises, named for Dr. John Kegel, who discovered them, can take a little practice before you isolate the correct muscles. Your doctor can teach you how to perform these exercises. There is also a helpful website that gives explicit directions: www.kegelexercisesforwomen.com.

If you've recently given birth, allow your body time to heal before engaging in sexual relations. Six weeks is the recommended amount of time. And at the other end of the spectrum, if menopause and its associated drop in estrogen levels is the cause of your pain, your physician can prescribe estrogen cream or ointment to help increase lubrication.

POINTERS ON PAIN

If you use a diaphragm, be sure it fits properly. This can be a simple fix to a painful problem.

Finally, if you've gone through the diagnostic procedures and nothing is helping, talking to a counselor can help you work through any issues you have concerning sex and sexual intercourse. Your physician can refer you to a mental health professional who specializes in this area.

Reproductive Tract Problems

The female reproductive tract consists of the uterus, ovaries, fallopian tubes, cervix, and vagina. Many pain issues in women center around these structures and pain can occur and recur on a monthly basis, as the body prepares for a possible pregnancy or cleanses itself of unneeded tissues when a pregnancy hasn't taken place.

Endometriosis

Your uterus has a lining, called the endometrium. Sometimes, for reasons not fully understood, this lining doesn't stay where it belongs, but instead grows on the ovaries, the fallopian tubes, or even over the tissue that lines the pelvis.

This tissue doesn't know it's not where it belongs, so it continues to behave as if it were in the right place. What this means for you is that each month the tissue thickens in preparation for a possible pregnancy. Because it's not located in the right place, after the thickening process is finished, the tissue then breaks down and sloughs. This sloughing is accomplished in your uterus with your monthly period. However, the endometrium doesn't have the proper outlet to let the blood flow from the uterus, so this blood stays confined in the wrong places.

 SPEAKING OF PAIN

It's estimated that more than five and a half million women in North America have endometriosis, and it's one of the top three causes of infertility in women.

The result is irritation, inflammation, and pain. Eventually adhesions can form, which adds to the pain.

Symptoms of endometriosis include extremely painful cramps during the menstrual period, along with heavy bleeding and chronic pelvic and intestinal pain. This pain may be so severe as to interfere with sexual relations.

You may have a genetic predisposition for developing endometriosis, since your risk factors for endometriosis increase if your mother had this condition. Other risk factors include the following:

- Menstrual cycle of fewer than 27 days accompanied with a period that lasts longer than 8 days

- Never having given birth

- Previous pelvic infection

Left untreated, endometriosis usually gets worse. Diagnosis includes evaluation of symptoms, physical examination that includes a pelvic exam, and diagnostic imaging tests such as ultrasound. Blood may be taken to look for a specific protein that is found in women with endometriosis.

Treatment may include both medications, such as nonsteroidal anti-inflammatory drugs (NSAIDs), hormone therapy, and laparoscopic surgery to remove excess tissue. In severe cases, hysterectomy may be indicated, although this ends any possibilities of future pregnancy.

POINTERS ON PAIN

Pelvic Congestion Syndrome is pain related to swollen veins that occurs outside the normal menstrual cycle and that lasts longer than six months.

Fibroid Disease of Uterus

Generally referred to as fibroids, these noncancerous tumors of the uterus are common. There seems to be a connection between their development and estrogen levels. These tumors continue to grow as long as an estrogen supply is available to feed them.

SPEAKING OF PAIN

Fibroids are found in about 20 percent of women during their childbearing years.

Chances are if there's one fibroid, there are more, and they come in all sizes, from microscopic to as big as an orange. Sometimes a fibroid isn't confined to the inside of the uterus, but instead develops on the outside, where it hangs from a stalk. This type of fibroid can cause sharp, severe pain.

Symptoms of fibroids include gas, increased frequency of urination, and a feeling of tightness or fullness in the lower abdomen and groin. You may experience bleeding between your periods as well, along with heavy cramping.

Diagnosis is made based upon your symptoms and a physical examination that includes a pelvic exam, along with an ultrasound of the pelvic area. In some cases a biopsy of the tissue is taken to rule out other conditions, such as cancer.

If you're not having symptoms, your physician may decide on a course of *expectant management*.

DEFINITION

Expectant management is the medical term for "watching and waiting." Your physician will monitor your fibroids, but treatment won't be initiated until symptoms warrant it.

If you are having symptoms, treatment may include NSAIDs, along with birth control pills to better regulate your menstrual periods and iron supplements to prevent anemia from loss of red blood cells. Your physician may decide that a course of hormone therapy to shrink the fibroids may be in order. This is not a permanent solution, however, and the fibroids are likely to regrow after hormone therapy is stopped.

If surgery is indicated, several different procedures can be done. A type of laparoscopic surgery, called hysteroscopic resection, can be done to remove fibroids growing inside the uterus. A myomectomy is a different procedure that also can remove intrauterine fibroids. If pregnancy is not a concern and the symptoms are severe, a hysterectomy can be performed.

POINTERS ON PAIN

The National Uterine Fibroid Foundation is an excellent resource for information on living with fibroids and treatment for them. Their website is www.nuff.org.

Premenstrual Syndrome

The onset of menstruation, called menarche, generally begins around the age of 12, although it can occur in younger girls as well. Each month after that, until menopause (the ceasing of menstruation that occurs generally between the ages of 45 to 50), a woman's body prepares for a possible pregnancy. During this time, the lining of the uterus thickens.

When a pregnancy doesn't take place, the uterus sheds this lining that becomes the monthly flow of blood, called the menses, and often referred to as "the period." The duration of the menses varies widely among women. It can last for just a couple of days or more than a week.

Some women experience mild discomfort during their periods, but for others this monthly experience can range from painful to incapacitating with symptoms that include nausea, vomiting, diarrhea, and backache. The medical term for painful periods is dysmenorrhea.

Risk factors for menstrual pain include some over which you have no control and some that you can control. Examples in the first category include having started your periods before the age of 11 and having those periods last longer than five days. You are more likely to have severe menstrual cramps if you have never been pregnant. Examples of risk factors that are within your control include smoking, alcohol consumption, and being overweight.

Menstrual cramps have a variety of causes. In some women, high levels of *prostaglandins* cause more intense uterine contractions, commonly referred to as cramps. They may also cause the nausea and other symptoms referred to previously.

DEFINITION

Prostaglandins are found throughout the body. They're hormonelike entities and are responsible for many different types of body functions.

Other causes may be endometriosis or fibroids (see previous sections), an ectopic pregnancy (see next section), infection, or an ovarian cyst. Some women experience menstrual pain if they are wearing an intrauterine device (IUD) for birth control.

Diagnosis is made based upon symptoms and a physical examination that includes a pelvic examination. In some cases, your doctor may order diagnostic imaging tests to see whether there are any abnormalities of the internal organs. These tests may include an ultrasound or a laparoscopy.

Treatment consists of NSAIDs, and they are more effective if you take them at the beginning of your period and continue them until your period has stopped.

A heating pad placed over the abdomen can be comforting. Be sure to wrap it in a protective cover or toweling to prevent burns to your skin.

Regular exercise can strengthen your abdominal muscles and decrease the severity of your cramping. If you're sedentary, talk to your physician before beginning an exercise regimen. After you get the go-ahead, make exercise part of your daily routine.

Often overlooked is the importance of a good diet, and that means one high in calcium and other essential vitamins and minerals. If your diet is sporadic in its healthiness, consider taking a daily multivitamin supplement.

Sometimes hormonal therapy is effective in relieving menstrual pain. Birth control pills may be prescribed for this purpose. Surgery is not generally indicated. In severe cases and when a future pregnancy is not desired, a hysterectomy can be performed to remove the uterus.

Ectopic Pregnancy

In an ectopic pregnancy, a fertilized egg attaches itself to an area outside the uterus. Usually this occurs on a fallopian tube, but it's possible for an ectopic pregnancy to occur in a variety of other places inside the abdomen.

In most cases, an ectopic pregnancy results when a blockage is in the fallopian tubes, generally because of prior surgery in this area or because of scar tissue due to an infection. In some cases, pelvic inflammatory disease is responsible for the scar tissue, but a strep or staph infection can also cause scarring in the abdominal cavity. Other causes of ectopic pregnancy are endometriosis or a congenital abnormality in the fallopian tubes.

SPEAKING OF PAIN

An ectopic pregnancy is not a normal pregnancy. Mortality rates for women with an ectopic pregnancy used to exceed 50 percent, but with advances in medical technology, the mortality rate has been significantly lowered.

Symptoms include low back pain, cramping, nausea, vaginal bleeding, and tenderness in the breasts. Any woman who is pregnant or could be pregnant should have these symptoms evaluated immediately. The danger with an ectopic pregnancy is that it can rupture, causing internal bleeding that can be extremely serious.

Diagnosis is made based upon an evaluation of symptoms, medical history, and a physical examination that includes a pelvic examination. Blood tests may be ordered that will detect pregnancy. In addition, diagnostic imaging tests may be used to confirm the diagnosis and find the exact source of the ectopic pregnancy.

Treatment for an ectopic pregnancy means surgically removing the implanted egg, which may mean removing the fallopian tube.

Pregnancy

During the nine months of a normal pregnancy, a woman's body undergoes many changes to accommodate the growing fetus. Tissues must stretch, hormone levels change, and fatigue and pain can be frequent annoyances. You're also more susceptible to urinary tract infections, inflammation of the pancreas, and gallbladder disease.

Minor problems, such as gas and constipation, can make you extremely uncomfortable. Seeking treatment early on for your symptoms can relieve your pain, heal any infection, and make your pregnancy more comfortable.

STABS AND JABS

Any vaginal bleeding during pregnancy should be evaluated by your physician. Do not wait for your regularly scheduled appointment.

Round Ligament Pain

Round ligament pain can occur on either or both sides of your abdomen, as well as in your groin area. Sometimes it's an annoying pull or ache, and other times it can feel as sharp as nerve pain. It's caused by the ligaments stretching as they must during your second trimester, if they are to continue to support your growing uterus.

Most often resting a bit will bring relief. If rest isn't helping, call your physician to see what she recommends.

POINTERS ON PAIN

During pregnancy, resist the urge to reach for any medications for pain relief, until you've checked with your physician. Side effects of some drugs may harm your fetus.

Joint and Back Pain

You'll most likely notice joint and back pain in the third trimester of pregnancy. The growing baby is getting heavier and as you go about your daily activities, your muscles, joints, and ligaments are getting a double workout. How you move can make a considerable difference in the level of that pain. Steps you can take include the following:

- Squatting to retrieve items on low shelves or to pick something up from the floor
- Switching to low-heeled shoes
- Resting whenever you can
- Sleeping on your side instead of your back
- Exercising according to your physician's recommendations
- Applying heating pads or ice packs where it hurts

If your pain worsens, or if you have any spotting or pink vaginal discharge, this may be a sign of early labor. Contact your physician at once.

Sacroiliac Joint Dysfunction

The sacroiliac joint is located at the base of your spine where it meets your pelvis. Prior to delivery, hormones are responsible for allowing this joint to loosen to prepare for birth. Excess movement or looseness of this joint has been linked to developing arthritis in that joint later in life.

Symptoms include pain in the lower back, although this pain can radiate outward to the buttocks, groin, or down the leg to the knee. Treatment is with NSAIDs and physical therapy to work at stabilizing and strengthening the muscles that support the joint. Surgery may be indicated if other treatments aren't effective.

Prevention

Regular exercise and a healthy diet are key to preventing many pain issues that center around the female experience. Moderate consumption of alcohol, along with not smoking, can also be helpful, and safer sex practices can prevent many of the infections that cause pain.

Treatment

From medications through counseling, treatment options are many and varied depending on the nature of the condition. Essential to each problem, however, is correct diagnosis, and for this your physician is the person to turn to.

The Least You Need to Know

- Painful menstruation is not a psychological problem but a treatable medical condition.
- Distinguishing the cause and proper course of treatment of vaginitis is a task for your doctor.
- An ectopic pregnancy is a medical emergency.
- Keeping physically fit during pregnancy can greatly reduce your risk of painful back and joint problems.

The Broader Picture of Pain

When pain becomes its own syndrome, it takes on a life of its own and treating it may require the expert hand of a pain specialist. Pain is also a symptom of many medical conditions. Often, pain is what gets you to make an appointment to see your doctor, and it's then that a diagnosis of the underlying medical condition can be discovered. After this is done, treatment for both the condition and the pain that it causes can begin. In Part 4, we'll examine the broader picture of pain.

Central Pain Syndrome

In This Chapter

- Sensory nerves and pain
- Deciding on a course of therapy
- Spinal cord injuries and pain
- The multidisciplinary approach to treating CPS

Central pain syndrome (CPS) is a neurological condition resulting from damage to the central nervous system (CNS). This syndrome can have several causes, ranging from trauma to an underlying medical condition, and the symptoms affect people in different ways. In this chapter, we'll explore the different causes of CPS, examine available treatments, and consider the prognosis.

When to See the Doctor

Because CPS develops after an injury or is a complication of an existing medical condition, you have one advantage: you're most likely seeing your doctor for the initial condition. This greatly helps in the diagnostic portion of dealing with CPS, since the trigger for the pain is often identified.

Diagnosis

CPS is a neurological condition that develops as a result of damage to the CNS. The damage doesn't necessarily destroy the nerve cells, but damages them to the point that they are unable to function normally.

Injured nerve cells don't transmit fewer impulses, but rather they transmit more of them. This malfunction eventually creates havoc with neighboring nerve cells, creating an avalanche of pain.

This syndrome can have several causes, ranging from trauma to an underlying medical condition. It's also known by several other names, including central poststroke syndrome, thalamic pain syndrome, and others.

CPS may occur as a result of multiple sclerosis, stroke, cancer, spinal cord injury, brain injury, or any of a variety of other medical conditions. Symptoms include pain typical of nerve pain: stabbing, sharp, or shooting. It can also manifest as a "pins and needles" or a dull, aching sensation.

Almost anything can trigger the pain—from the lightest touch (which can include human touch or the weight of a bed sheet) to a change in the barometric pressure.

The nervous system is complex. Your body has motor nerves and sensory nerves. The former carry impulses from your CNS to your muscles, telling them how to move, when to move, where to move, and when to stop moving. When motor nerves become injured, they can impede your ability to move normally.

Sensory nerves have a different purpose. They relay information to the CNS and vice versa. An example mentioned in a previous chapter can illustrate how this works. Suppose you touch a hot pan on the stove. That act begins the sensory nerve relay process.

In less than a second, those sensory nerves relay the information that your fingers are burning. The brain receives that information through the spinal cord and decides the best course of action is to drop that pot. You do, and mission accomplished. You tend to the burn, it heals, and all is well.

When these sensory nerves are injured, however, they don't function this way. They don't function normally. To make matters worse, the motor nerves can also become overstimulated. Nothing works the way it's supposed to.

There seems to be a short circuit of sorts with nerve injury. It's almost as if they become hysterical—screaming their pain message at a frantic pace over and over, and continuing with this intense message long after you've dropped the pot that burned your fingers and the burn has healed.

The damaged nerves simply don't give up. These sensory nerves cannot distinguish between the lightest touch and the sharpest blow. Their message-sending capabilities have become distorted. Symptoms include the characteristic nerve pain: sharp and burning. Other symptoms include the following:

- Pain that gets worse with movement or with touch

- Extreme painful sensitivity to cold

- Ineffectiveness of pain relievers

Diagnosis is made based upon symptoms and medical history. Diagnostic imaging tests are not always effective in diagnosing this condition. Your physician may refer you to a neurologic pain specialist for treatment. The following sections discuss some of the medical conditions that can lead to CPS.

Poststroke Pain

A stroke results when some portion of the brain is deprived of its blood supply. Blood carries oxygen, which the brain needs to survive. Without the oxygen, brain cells die. The more serious the stroke, the more brain cells are affected. It takes only a few minutes for serious or fatal consequences to develop after a stroke, so immediate emergency medical care is necessary to prevent death or long-term disability.

Chronic nerve pain, called central poststroke pain, can result in the aftermath of a stroke. Symptoms can begin almost immediately or not develop for some time, but after this pain begins, it doesn't go away. Because it's nerve pain, it can be burning and sharp. The pain occurs along the side of the body affected by the stroke and can involve the arm, side, leg, and face.

POINTERS ON PAIN

Central poststroke pain is more likely to develop if the stroke has occurred on the right side of the brain.

Preventing poststroke pain means preventing a stroke from happening in the first place. Prevention involves reducing risk factors such as high blood pressure and high cholesterol. You can't control your genetics, but you can adopt a healthy lifestyle and give yourself every possible advantage. Some things you can do include the following:

- Quitting smoking

- Lowering high cholesterol

- Reducing high blood pressure

- Drinking in moderation

- Eating a healthy diet

- Exercising regularly

When diet and exercise aren't sufficient to keep your blood pressure and cholesterol down, your physician can prescribe medication to help you achieve good numbers. Here's how those good numbers translate.

You're probably familiar with the procedure for taking your blood pressure, but the numbers resulting from this simple, routine procedure may be confusing. A blood pressure reading consists of two numbers. The first number, called the systolic pressure, is the pressure when your heart contracts. The second number, called the dystolic pressure, is the pressure when your heart relaxes. The numbers are written with the systolic pressure over the dystolic pressure. A normal blood pressure reading is 120/80.

If your numbers are too high, you are at risk for a heart attack or a stroke and medication may be needed to bring them back down to acceptable limits.

Your cholesterol is also reported with two numbers that, when added together, should not exceed 200. The first is your HDL (you want this high, so think H = high). The second is your LDL (you want this low, so think L = low). Another cholesterol measurement checks your triglyceride level. You want this reading to be under 150. If your cholesterol levels are too high, medication may be necessary to bring them under control.

If you have coronary artery disease or diabetes, you are at increased risk for stroke. See your physician regularly to be sure you are managing these conditions to the best of your ability.

The sooner medical treatment for a stroke can begin, the better the chances for recovery. Immediate emergency medical care is essential. Clot-buster drugs can be administered by injection or intravenously to quickly open up the blocked artery and restore blood flow. Time is of the essence, however, and these drugs must be given shortly after the stroke in order to be effective.

Two courses of therapy are involved: one is focused on treating the stroke and the other on managing poststroke pain. Treatment of stroke may include blood thinners, such as heparin or aspirin, along with blood pressure medications to reduce the risk of additional stroke. Medications include oral medications, such as amitriptyline, along with anticonvulsants and antidepressants.

Nerve blocks, deep brain stimulation, and motor cortex stimulation have produced good results for treating poststroke pain in about half of those undergoing the procedure. Injection of anesthetics to inhibit nerve impulses is also a treatment option. In addition, learning techniques for managing stress can relieve tension—a prime contributor to the intensity of the pain you feel.

Parkinson's Disease

Parkinson's disease causes changes in nerve cells in the brain. These changes alter the way the brain produces a specific chemical (dopamine) that is responsible for movement. As a result, your brain produces less dopamine, and you have difficulty controlling how your body moves—your body doesn't do what you want it to.

Changes in muscle movement can cause many different types of pain. Parkinson's is a chronic condition that is progressive, which means there's no cure, and symptoms can worsen over time. Fortunately, many treatments are available to help you manage Parkinson's.

SPEAKING OF PAIN

It is estimated that about 40 percent of people with Parkinson's experience some type of associated pain.

Pain associated with Parkinson's can affect the shoulders, neck, and back, and often the legs as well. This pain is usually caused by tight muscles and loss of range of motion in the joints. A compounding problem is that since it hurts to move, you tend to move less, which makes the situation worse.

Symptoms include generalized aches that can be more intense during periods of dystonia. Many types of pain are associated with Parkinson's—ranging from mild aching muscles to sharp, burning nerve pain.

In addition to the muscle and joint pain from lack of movement, Parkinson's disease also causes central pain. Like other causes of central pain, you can feel general sensations of burning, shooting, and stabbing pain all over the body. This pain is not relieved with changes in position or with movement.

DEFINITION

Dystonia refers to the spasms felt in parts of the feet and the hands. For example, ankles or fingers may twist into uncomfortable positions; the feeling is one of cramping.

Because Parkinson's affects the production of dopamine in the brain, medications are used to slow the loss of dopamine. These medications include the following:

- Levodopa
- Sinemet
- Requip
- Mirapex
- Parlodel
- Permax
- Eldepryl or Deprenyl

Antidepressants can also be used to manage neuropathic pain by either increasing the dopamine or decreasing the rate of its loss.

It can take time to determine the right medications and the right dosages to manage your Parkinson's pain. Many of these medications have adverse side effects, so be sure to tell your doctor whether you're experiencing an increase in symptoms or notice any changes in your condition.

In addition, prescription and over-the-counter pain relievers, heating pads, and physical therapy can help restore some flexibility and range of movement. Managing CPS in Parkinson's disease is a team effort. Your primary care physician and a pain medicine specialist can develop a treatment protocol to help you achieve maximum relief from your pain.

STABS AND JABS

Depression is a common companion to chronic disease, and it's a serious complication. Treatments are available for depression, so check with your physician and give yourself the strength to cope.

Cancer

When cancer infects the spinal cord or brain, CPS can develop as a result. The cause may be traced to the cancer, chemotherapy or radiation used to treat the cancer, or there may another cause that cannot be identified.

One of the problems is that recent advances in treatment have extended the life span of many individuals with cancer, but these treatments may have adverse effects on the quality of that life. CPS is one of those adverse effects.

Medications implicated in the development of CPS and other nerve pain problems such as neuropathies include the following:

- Cisplatin (Platinol)
- Vincristine
- Ifosfamide (Ifex)
- Paclitaxel

Individuals with pre-existing neuropathy may find themselves at greater risk for developing CPS after chemotherapy. Corticosteroids may be helpful in treating CPS in individuals with CNS cancer. One medication in particular, dexamethasone, has been useful in this regard.

Additionally, local anesthetics such as lidocaine have also been reported to have given some relief from pain.

Anticonvulsants and antidepressants have been effective in some instances, but much research remains to be done in this area.

Multiple Sclerosis

Multiple sclerosis (MS) is an autoimmune disease that causes scarring throughout the CNS, which consists of the brain and the spinal cord. This scarring, called sclerosis, occurs in multiple places, hence the name multiple sclerosis. Chronic pain is experienced by nearly half of those affected with multiple sclerosis.

The National Multiple Sclerosis Society reports that as many as 400,000 adults in the United States have MS, with women affected three times more often than men.

Excluding traumatic injuries, MS is the most common cause of neurological disability in adults through middle age.

Eye pain is a common problem with MS, and it can be an early diagnostic clue to the presence of this condition. The optic nerve can become inflamed, a condition referred to as optic neuritis.

POINTERS ON PAIN

Sometimes you can fool damaged nerves and change what they sense as pain into pressure or warmth. Wear a pressure glove or stocking and try warm compresses on painful skin areas.

With MS, pain can occur throughout the body. A stabbing pain in the face, called trigeminal neuralgia, can come on with various facial movements. Anything from chewing to sneezing can cause an attack. Even a slight touch on the face can cause pain, and hygiene becomes a test of strength, as brushing your teeth can lead to sharp pain in your face. Other body movements, such as bending forward from the waist, can also trigger nerve pain.

Nonsteroidal anti-inflammatory drugs (NSAIDs) don't provide much help in relieving the pain of MS, since the source isn't muscle fatigue or joint problems. Though patients with MS can also have muscle and joint pain from inability to move properly, if the source of pain is neurological, NSAIDs will not be useful. To tease out the causes of pain, a trial of NSAIDs may be given.

Anticonvulsant medications, such as Tegretol and Neurontin, have been used with some benefit. These medications haven't received official endorsement by the FDA for use in managing pain.

POINTERS ON PAIN

Botox, the same treatment used to repair facial wrinkles, may show some promise as a means of providing pain relief in MS. Research into its use is ongoing.

Spinal Cord Injuries

The spinal cord is the link between the brain and the body's nerve cells. It transmits information constantly and is responsible for your body's ability to react and to move.

When the spinal cord is injured, this transmission gets interrupted. In some cases, the interruption is permanent, and paralysis can occur.

> ☞ **SPEAKING OF PAIN**
>
> It is estimated that up to 85 percent of those with spinal cord injuries will develop CPS.

Falls, motor vehicle accidents, and violence are the primary causes of spinal cord injuries, although certain medical conditions such as spina bifida (in which the spine doesn't fully develop), arthritis, or severe cervical stenosis may also be responsible. However, the medical causes make up less than 10 percent of all spinal cord injuries in the United States.

Both acute and chronic pain can accompany spinal cord injuries. Within these two broad categories can be different types and levels of pain. There is also an emotional trauma associated with a new spinal cord injury that of course makes any kind of pain worse.

There are many causes for immediate pain for patients with spinal cord injuries. This acute course can include pain from ulcers to the skin, broken bones, and ruptured joints. The pain comes on with the injury. When the pain doesn't resolve, it can become its own entity—called chronic pain. Chronic pain can involve the nerves (neuropathic), the bones and muscles (musculoskeletal), or the internal organs (visceral). Basically, any pain that lasts longer than one month can be considered chronic.

Neuropathic pain can be burning, sharp, and stabbing in nature, and is common after a spinal cord injury. This pain may not develop immediately after an injury but may take weeks or even months to come on. Some nerve pain is felt at the site of the injury or just above or below the site. It can hurt even if you've lost sensation in the area.

> **POINTERS ON PAIN**
>
> Changes in temperature or even a light touch can create painful sensations in the skin near the site of a spinal cord injury. This heightened sensitivity is called allodynia.

Other nerve pain can occur just at the spot where sensation changes—at the boundary between loss of sensation and normal sensation. Any touch can aggravate this pain, which is called nerve root entrapment pain and is caused by compression of a nerve root at a joint or between pieces of bone.

Musculoskeletal pain is usually less sharp and stabbing than nerve pain. Joints and muscles ache either because of spasms that occur as a result of damaged nerves that transmit corrupted nerve signals, or because you compensate for loss of function in one part of the body by overusing other, functional parts.

Visceral pain is internal. It's felt in the abdomen as cramping or burning and tends to become chronic.

Treatment of spinal cord injury pain is challenging. A combination of medications, physical therapy, and surgery can help relieve the pain, although totally eliminating it may not be possible. Medications may include Neurontin, amitriptyline, or nortriptyline. A pain pump is another option that has been helpful in many cases. Other options include the following:

- Spinal cord stimulation

- Nerve blocks

- Decompression surgery

A physical or occupational therapist can help you manage pain resulting from overuse of certain muscles in one area to compensate for loss of movement in another.

Often, deciding to give up this overuse of functioning body parts is an intensely emotional experience. Deciding that a power chair may be easier on your shoulders than a manual chair, for example, is coupled with a realization of loss of control.

The psychological aspects of spinal cord injury are as real and as painful as any associated with CPS. Working with a mental health professional, as well as with occupational and physical therapists, can help you cope with these changes.

Prevention

The only prevention for CPS is preventing the medical condition or trauma that leads to its development. In some cases where the cause isn't known, prevention isn't possible.

In other cases, such as stroke or trauma, some preventive measures do exist. Reducing your risk of coronary artery disease is the prime measure for preventing stroke. Guarding against accidents to the best of your ability is always a good plan, but accidents do happen, and in many cases they aren't your fault. All you can do is the best you can do.

Treatment

CPS is usually treated with anticonvulsant and antidepressant medications, both of which have the capacity to relieve pain. It can take some time to arrive at the right combination and dosage of these medications. In severe cases, narcotics may be indicated, and surgery to implant a pain pump or for deep brain stimulation may be necessary to relieve the pain.

When the pain cannot be managed by medication or with an implant, in some instances you can opt for surgery to sever the affected nerves, although in the majority of cases the pain does recur in a different location.

The psychological aspects of living with CPS can be considerable, and using a multidisciplinary approach to pain management is often the best course of action. Your team may include your primary care physician, neurologist, physical and occupational therapists, and a mental health professional, such as a psychotherapist.

A psychotherapist can provide training in cognitive behavior therapy, which can be helpful in learning coping strategies for living with this condition. Your physician or neurologist can refer you to a psychotherapist.

Living with CPS is not easy. Living with any chronic, painful condition can lead to depression. You may begin to feel that it's not worth the struggle and may feel that your prognosis is grim. If these feelings continue for more than two weeks, talk to your doctor about them. In some cases, depression is a side effect of medications. Changing your dosage or switching to a different medication may resolve the problem.

Depression is real. It's an identifiable medical condition, and it can be treated. If changes in your medications don't provide relief, your physician can refer you to a mental health professional who will help you learn how to manage pain so it doesn't manage you.

In addition to counseling, try some self-empowerment strategies (see Chapter 8). And finally, whatever the condition you have that's responsible for CPS, there's a support group of people like you who can offer advice, humor, and encouragement. You can find one through your local hospital or check online through your medical condition's website.

The Least You Need to Know

- CPS develops when the nervous system, including the brain and spinal cord, is damaged.
- Antidepressants and anticonvulsant medications may be helpful in managing the pain of CPS.
- CPS can develop shortly after a trauma or the onset of a medical condition or may take years to manifest.
- Treating CPS requires a multidisciplinary approach.
- Treating depression associated with CPS will help you manage your pain.

Pain Related to Other Medical Conditions

In This Chapter

- Managing arthritis pain
- Preventing type 2 diabetes
- Blood vessels and pain
- Coping with cancer pain

Pain is a symptom of injury or illness. When it's a symptom of illness, sometimes treating that illness relieves the pain. When treating the illness doesn't cause the pain to go away and the pain becomes chronic, it then becomes a medical condition of its own, and treatment becomes more challenging. In this chapter, we'll take a look at a variety of medical conditions that can cause pain and explore your options for getting relief.

When to See the Doctor

Pain is a symptom of many medical conditions. If you have been managing your pain symptoms but the frequency, duration, or type of pain has changed, it's important to check with your doctor. Sometimes an adjustment in the type or dosage of your medications is all that's needed to solve the problem. Other times, the pain may be serving as your body's early warning system that something more serious is amiss, especially if the pain comes on suddenly. The bottom line: Don't try to be your own diagnostician. When you have pain and are concerned, talk to your doctor.

Diagnosis

Perhaps the most important component of a diagnosis here is your medical history. Your symptoms of pain by themselves don't necessarily offer enough information, but a physical examination along with an analysis of your medical history can provide the clues as to the source of your pain. With the addition of blood work and diagnostic imaging tests, your physician can get to the source of the problem, and you can begin to get relief from your pain.

Arthritis

Arthritis is something we're all familiar with. If you don't have arthritis, it's fairly certain that a friend or family member does. Arthritis means "inflammation of the joint." It's a broad term, and although not all types of arthritis involve an inflammatory response, some do. The two types of arthritis people are most familiar with are osteoarthritis and rheumatoid arthritis, but many other conditions are lumped under the category of arthritis. One aspect they all share, however, is pain.

Osteoarthritis

This is the wear-and-tear type of arthritis and the most common form. It develops over time, as the cartilage that cushions your joints becomes repeatedly overused and worn out. This chronic degeneration causes the cartilage to become stiff instead of rubbery, and it loses its ability to protect the bones in the joint. Osteoarthritis (OA) is not an inflammatory type of arthritis.

> **SPEAKING OF PAIN**
>
> In the United States alone, more than 21 million people have osteoarthritis. That number is magnified millions of times over, when you consider its impact on the worldwide population.

With the cartilage not functioning, there's a ripple effect. Ligaments don't fit as well, and the ends of the bones can overgrow, developing bone spurs. The result of the ripple effect is pain, as bone grinds against bone. Symptoms of osteoarthritis include pain, stiffness, and loss of mobility in the affected joint. Hips, spine, knees, wrists, hands, thumbs, ankles, and feet are common sites for OA.

Risk factors for developing OA include being overweight, overusing a joint, being an adult over the age of 40, having had a prior injury to a joint, or having other family members with OA—the genetic connection. The first two factors are the only ones over which you have some degree of control.

Diagnosis is based upon symptoms, physical examination, and diagnostic imaging tests, such as x-rays or an MRI.

There is no cure for OA, but there is help to manage the pain it causes. Treatment of OA will depend upon how severe your symptoms are. Your physician will recommend a program of active rest. That means resting your joints when they hurt and engaging in regular, low-impact aerobic exercise when they don't. A physical therapist can guide you through a program of strengthening and flexibility exercises.

POINTERS ON PAIN

Walking is the simplest, cheapest, and easiest form of low-impact aerobic exercise.

Over-the-counter and prescription medications can help relieve the pain of OA. Your physician may prescribe acetaminophen (Tylenol) for mild symptoms, along with a topical ointment or cream. More severe pain may require injections of steroids directly into the joint. In some cases, joint replacement surgery may be a good option.

Lifestyle changes are not always easy, but if you are overweight, you're putting extra stress on already overtaxed joints. Losing weight decreases that stress. If you have OA, maintaining a proper weight can significantly lessen your pain and may help prevent OA from developing in certain joints. Your doctor will tell you that losing weight is the number-one action you can take to relieve the pain of OA.

Overuse of your joints doesn't just mean misusing them. If your occupation requires you to bend, stoop, lift, or perform other repetitive joint motions, your joints may eventually reach their maximum capability to absorb stress. Prevention here means finding alternative ways to perform your tasks that don't put so much wear and tear on your joints. Sometimes that's not possible, and that can mean retraining for a different position or even changing your line of work in order to protect your body.

Rheumatoid Arthritis

Rheumatoid arthritis (RA) is an *autoimmune disease* and a form of inflammatory arthritis that attacks the lining of the joints, causing that lining to become inflamed and swollen. Over time, this inflammation spreads to the joints, and eventually the joints themselves become misshapen and painful.

DEFINITION

An **autoimmune disease** is one in which the body's immune system malfunctions and decides that the body is an invader, instead of the entity it is supposed to protect. In the case of RA, the immune system targets the joint lining, eventually destroying it.

Most often RA begins in the smaller joints, such as the fingers. It tends to be symmetrical, meaning that the same parts on both sides of the body are affected. Common symptoms of RA include joint pain and swelling around the joint. Other symptoms include the following:

- Stiffness in the morning lasting more than one hour
- Weight loss and decreased appetite
- Fatigue
- Lack of energy

RA can also affect the organs, and so it is called a systemic disease. You may feel pain in your chest. If this happens when you breathe, your lungs may have become involved. If you notice pain in your chest when you move about, it may be a sign that the tissues surrounding the heart have become inflamed.

Diagnosis is made based upon symptoms, physical examination, blood work, and diagnostic imaging tests. The presence of an antibody called rheumatoid factor (RF) and an antibody called Anti-CCP in your blood are good diagnostic clues for RA.

SPEAKING OF PAIN

About 1.3 million Americans have rheumatoid arthritis, of which 75 percent are women.

Your physician may use a needle and a syringe to remove some fluid from one of the affected joints to send to the lab for analysis. This is called joint fluid aspiration or arthrocentesis. This is both a diagnostic tool and a treatment, since removing some fluid from the joint can relieve the pressure and the accompanying pain.

Treatment for RA has several components. It includes nonsteroidal anti-inflammatory drugs (NSAIDs), low-dose corticosteroids, a new class of medications called disease-modifying antirheumatic drugs (DMARDs), and another class of medications called biologic response modifiers (biologics).

Rest, exercise, and physical therapy are also recommended to help you increase flexibility and maintain or restore range of motion in your joints. In severe cases that don't respond to treatment, joint replacement surgery may be indicated.

Psoriatic Arthritis

Psoriatic arthritis is a type of inflammatory arthritis that can accompany psoriasis. Psoriatic arthritis can take different forms, and symptoms vary depending upon which form you have. The greatest risk factor for developing psoriatic arthritis is having psoriasis. Other risk factors include a prior strep infection, stress, poor diet, alcohol abuse, or skin injuries. Psoriatic arthritis can also develop as a reaction to medications or vaccinations.

Diagnosis of psoriatic arthritis can be difficult, since you have to have symptoms of both psoriasis and arthritis present at the same time. Either condition can develop first. When this happens, treatment can begin.

Treatment includes NSAIDs, or a COX-2 inhibitor (Celebrex) to relieve pain, swelling, and stiffness. Other medications include any of the disease-modifying antirheumatics, such as sulfasalazine, Plaquenil, and methotrexate. Slowing the rate of joint damage with tumor necrosis factor (TNF) blockers is important.

Infectious Arthritis

Infectious arthritis is also known as septic arthritis. The name is a bit misleading, since the condition is not contagious. In infectious arthritis, some type of microbe (such as a fungus, virus, or bacteria) gains entrance to a joint and begins to multiply.

Risk factors for developing infectious arthritis include the following:

- Having a suppressed immune system
- Previous injury or surgery to a joint
- Underlying medical conditions, such as diabetes or sickle cell disease, or any rheumatologic condition
- History of intravenous (IV) drug abuse

Symptoms include joint pain and inflammation (swelling, warmth, tenderness, redness), along with fever or chills.

Infectious arthritis is diagnosed based upon symptoms, physical examination, blood work, and analysis of joint fluid drawn from the affected joint.

Treatment consists of draining the infected fluid from the joint and a course of antibiotics, targeted at the particular microbe that is causing the problem. Treatment must begin quickly, before permanent damage to the joint occurs.

Gout and Pseudogout

On a pain scale of 1 to 10, gout sometimes feels like an 11. Both gout and pseudogout are forms of *crystalline arthritis*, although the crystals involved are different. Uric acid crystals are responsible for gout, and calcium pyrophosphate crystals are responsible for pseudogout, which frequently affects the knee.

DEFINITION

Crystalline arthritis is the term given to types of arthritis in which certain types of crystals manufactured by the body deposit in the joint, causing inflammation and pain. Gout and pseudogout are common forms of crystalline arthritis.

Symptoms of gout are severe pain, usually in the joint below the big toe. Although other joints (generally in the foot or ankle) can be affected, the classic manifestation of gout is in the big toe. The joint is swollen, red, and shiny, and even the gentlest touch or the smallest movement intensifies the already excruciating pain.

Risk factors for gout include a genetic predisposition (heredity), obesity, a diet high in fats and low in fiber, consumption of seafood, and overindulgence in alcohol.

Diagnosis is made based upon symptoms, physical examination, and blood work to see whether you have elevated levels of uric acid.

One attack of gout may predispose you to future ones. Prevention centers around addressing your risk factors. Again, you can't control your genetics, but you can control your diet. If you're overweight, losing the extra pounds and keeping them off by switching to a low-fat, high-fiber diet will go a long way toward keeping your feet healthy.

Treatment involves resting your painful foot, and elevating it can bring some relief. NSAIDs can help with both pain and inflammation. Your physician may prescribe corticosteroid as an oral medication or inject it into the joint. Other prescription medications, such as colchicine to treat an initial attack, and probenecid or sulfin-pyraxone to lower uric acid levels over the long term, may be indicated.

Pseudogout usually targets the knee, although like gout it can affect other joints as well. It may be associated with the aging process, and may also have a genetic component.

> **SPEAKING OF PAIN**
>
> Pseudogout is generally a condition affecting older people. A typical pseudo-gout patient is 70 years old. Almost half of those with pseudogout are 85 and older.

Diagnosis of pseudogout is similar to that of gout, although the treatment plan differs, since the crystal deposit is different.

NSAIDs are often prescribed, and injection of a corticosteroid into the affected joint can be helpful. Regular, moderate, low-impact aerobic exercise can strengthen the muscles around the affected joint, and application of hot and cold packs can also relieve the pain.

Generalized Nerve Disorders

In some medical conditions, such as diabetes and fibromyalgia, pain can be felt throughout the body. Sometimes the targeted area is the peripheral nerves, found in the hands and feet. This is a common symptom of diabetes. Sometimes the pain seems to be everywhere at once. Everything hurts, and you can't isolate one particular part of your body as the source. This is a common symptom of fibromyalgia.

Diabetes

In broad terms, diabetes is a malfunctioning of the body's metabolic system. Glucose, a form of sugar, is used by the body's cells as their energy source. Glucose comes from the foods you eat and requires insulin to move it into the cells of your bloodstream. This insulin is produced by your pancreas. Usually, the right amount of insulin is produced, your cells get the necessary amounts of glucose, and your body is nourished.

> **SPEAKING OF PAIN**
>
> According to the National Diabetes Information Clearinghouse, around 24 million Americans have diabetes, and if you're obese, your chance of developing adult-onset type 2 diabetes increases threefold.

Sometimes the pancreas doesn't produce enough insulin to get the job done, and sometimes it doesn't produce any at all. When this happens, glucose levels build up in the bloodstream instead of moving into the cells. The glucose then passes out of your body in your urine as a waste product instead of being utilized as an energy source.

There are three common forms of diabetes:

1. Type 1 diabetes is an autoimmune disease in which the immune system attacks the pancreas, destroying the insulin-producing cells. This type requires daily injections of insulin.

2. Type 2 diabetes is also known as adult-onset diabetes. In many cases, this is a lifestyle-caused medical condition and can be prevented.

3. Gestational diabetes occurs during the later stages of pregnancy in some women and can predispose them to later developing type 2 diabetes.

Without nourishment, small blood vessels die. These blood vessels carry oxygen and other nutrients to the central nervous system (CNS), and without this nourishment the nerves suffer damage, and damaged nerves send pain signals.

Symptoms of type 1 diabetes include intense thirst, frequent urination, extreme hunger coupled with weight loss, fatigue, and irritability. Symptoms of type 2 diabetes include these symptoms along with blurred vision, frequent infections, skin injuries (cuts or bruises) that take a long time to heal, tingling or numbness in the hands and/or feet, and recurring infections of skin, bladder, or gums.

> **STABS AND JABS**
>
> Many times people with type 2 diabetes have no early symptoms. That's why it's important to have that annual physical examination.

Diagnosis is made based upon symptoms, medical history, and urinalysis. The fasting blood glucose test is the specific test run on the urine sample. A reading of 126 or above is an indicator for diabetes.

Type 1 diabetes is not preventable at this time, but type 2 diabetes can often be prevented with healthy lifestyle changes. These include regular exercise and a diet high in fiber and whole grains and low in fats.

If adopting a healthier lifestyle through diet and exercise isn't enough to prevent type 2 diabetes, medications can be added to your regimen. These include the following:

- Alpha-glucosidase inhibitors
- Sulonylureas and meglitinides
- Biguanides
- DPP-4 inhibitors
- Thiazolidinediones

Complications of diabetes are serious, so it's important to manage your blood sugar levels. This will give you the best chance of avoiding these complications, which include peripheral neuropathy—nerve pain that can be intense. This pain is generally felt first in your feet.

Treatment of peripheral neuropathy requires that blood sugar levels be brought back under control. Regular foot checks are necessary to tend to any cuts and infections, since numbness may keep you from noticing these types of injuries. Medications for the pain include analgesics, along with antidepressants and anticonvulsants.

Fibromyalgia

Although fatigue may be the first symptom you notice with fibromyalgia, pain is close on its heels. This is full-body pain and results from "haywiring of the brain." This aching pain may affect the muscles and the ligaments and tendons associated with the muscles, and at times, even the lightest touch can hurt. Tender points are symptomatic of fibromyalgia. They occur in various places on your body and extend from the back of your head all the way to your inner knees.

Fibromyalgia is often found in people who have another medical condition, such as irritable bowel syndrome (IBS) or any of several of the rheumatologic conditions. Fibromyalgia is more common in women.

Diagnosis of fibromyalgia is based upon two symptoms as specified by the American College of Rheumatology. You must have pain that is widespread over your body for at least three months. This is the generally recognized point at which acute pain becomes chronic. The other symptom centers around those tender points mentioned earlier. There are 18 of them, and during your physical examination, 11 or more of these tender points must be tender to the touch.

Treatment includes NSAIDs, anticonvulsants, and antidepressants. You may be referred to a physical therapist to begin a program of exercise designed to increase your muscle strength and endurance.

Because stress increases the perception of pain, cognitive behavioral therapy may be a good option for learning to manage stress. Your physician can refer you to a psychotherapist trained in cognitive behavioral therapy.

"Fibro fog" is a common symptom of fibromyalgia and speaks to the psychological pain and suffering this medical condition can cause. Essentially, your brain opts out at the most embarrassing and inconvenient times and it does so in a multitude of ways. For example:

- You may start a sentence and forget where you were going with your idea.

- You may find yourself with a pen in your hand and wonder why you're holding it.

- You may repeat yourself during a conversation and wonder why you're getting strange looks from your conversational partner.

The examples go on and on, but they're very real to someone with fibromyalgia. The problem is physiological, not psychological, but that can be small comfort. Symptoms can increase when your sleep is disturbed, and disturbed sleep patterns are a classic symptom of fibromyalgia. Practice sleep hygiene and discuss ways to improve the quality of your sleep with your physician to help reduce fibro fog's impact on your life.

Vascular Disease and Pain

Vascular disease refers to any disease that develops in the circulatory system outside the heart. Blood disorders that affect the arteries, veins, and other blood vessels fall into this category. These disorders include clots, *aneurysms*, arterial spasms, and varicose veins.

 DEFINITION

An **aneurysm** is an abnormal, localized widening of a blood vessel. This results in a bulge that weakens the wall of the blood vessel. An aneurysm can burst at any time and is life-threatening.

Sickle Cell Disease

Sickle cell disease is a genetically transmitted blood disorder that affects the hemoglobin. It's found most often in people of African descent. It gets its name from the distorted sickle- or scythelike shape the diseased hemoglobin molecules assume as they group together, instead of moving freely about the blood vessels as they are supposed to. These sickled cells block the blood vessels, and that blockage stops the flow of blood that's carrying oxygen and other nutrients throughout the body.

SPEAKING OF PAIN

It is estimated that about two million African Americans in the United States have sickle cell disease, with the incidence occurring once in every 500 births.

The sickled cells have a much-shortened life span and die off quickly. Since fewer healthy red blood cells are left in the body, anemia (a low red blood cell count) can develop, the most common symptom of sickle cell disease.

The blockage created by the sickled cells causes pain, referred to as a sickle crisis or a pain crisis. This pain often occurs in the arms, legs, and chest in adults, and in young children occurs frequently in the fingers and toes. Complications of sickle cell disease can include stroke, jaundice, and lung damage.

Diagnosis is made based upon symptoms, medical history, physical examination, and blood work. A specific blood test called a hemoglobin electrophoresis test can detect whether an individual is carrying the specific sickle cell gene.

Treatment includes NSAIDs, increased water intake to prevent or treat sickle crisis, penicillin to treat or prevent infection, and folic acid for anemia. In some cases of severe sickle cell disease, a bone marrow transplant may provide a cure, but as with all types of surgery, significant risks must be considered first.

Deep Venous Thrombosis

You may not be familiar with the medical terminology, but if you do any traveling, you're well aware of this condition. The common term is a blood clot in the vein. Deep venous thrombosis (DVT) is most common in older adults, but it can develop in individuals of any age.

Because traveling involves long periods of sitting, blood flow in your legs can be restricted, so it's recommended you get up and stretch frequently or do leg exercises if you must remain seated to prevent a clot from forming. Although the clot itself may cause pain, if the clot breaks free, it can travel through the bloodstream to the lungs, heart, brain, or other places and be life-threatening.

Risk factors include smoking, being confined to bed, sitting for long periods of time, fractures, having had recent surgery, or having given birth within the previous six months. Some medications, such as estrogen and birth control pills, and certain medical conditions, such as polycythemia vera or cancer, can increase your risk for deep venous thrombosis.

Symptoms include pain, swelling, redness, warmth, or tenderness in a leg. Diagnosis is made based upon symptoms, physical examination, blood work, and diagnostic imaging tests such as ultrasound.

Treatment is with anticoagulant medications. Initially these dissolve the clot and are later used to prevent formation of future clots. If medications aren't successful, surgery to remove the clot may be indicated.

Peripheral Artery Disease

Peripheral artery disease (PAD) is the most common form of vascular disease. It generally affects the arteries in the pelvis and the legs and has much in common with coronary artery disease. The primary symptom is a cramping pain in the legs when you're walking, exercising, or climbing.

Diagnosis is made based upon symptoms, medical history, and a physical examination that includes a specific test that measures the blood pressure in your feet and compares it to the blood pressure in your arm. In PAD, the blood flow is restricted, which affects your blood pressure. To confirm the diagnosis, your physician may recommend diagnostic imaging tests.

Treatment centers around positive lifestyle changes, which include regular low-impact aerobic exercise, along with a diet high in fiber and low in saturated and trans fats. If you smoke, you're advised to quit. The American Heart Association notes that smokers have four times the risk of developing PAD than do nonsmokers.

Medications to lower blood pressure and cholesterol, along with antiplatelet medications, may be prescribed. In some cases, surgery may be indicated to remove a clot or place a stent in the vein that's blocked.

Cancer

Cancer can cause pain on more than one level. First of all, the disease itself can cause pain, as it destroys tissue. If the cancer metastasizes (spreads), the pain spreads with it. Tumors, which are abnormal overgrowths of cells, can press upon nerves, causing sharp, shooting pain. If the tumors press upon bones or muscles, the pain may be more aching.

SPEAKING OF PAIN

It is estimated that up to half of people with cancer have pain symptoms at some time, and up to 90 percent of those with advanced cancer experience pain. Fortunately, most cases of pain can be successfully managed.

Cancer pain can become chronic as the disease progresses. Sometimes pain that has been previously successfully managed with medication "breaks through" this wall of therapy. This breakthrough pain can be difficult to treat.

The treatments for cancer can also be sources of pain. Surgery, chemotherapy, and radiation are not without side effects, and one of them, of course, is pain. Medications used in treating pain associated with cancer include the following:

- Analgesics (pain relievers such as aspirin or acetaminophen)

- NSAIDs, such as naproxen and ibuprofen

- Opioids, such as codeine, morphine, or oxycodone

These medications are available as tablets, through injection, or delivered intravenously. In addition, nerve blocks may provide relief from chronic pain, and self-help strategies can be useful tools for coping when the pain can't be totally controlled. See Chapter 8 for a discussion of these strategies.

The Least You Need to Know

- Maintaining a proper weight is the best way to both treat and prevent arthritis pain.
- Type 2 diabetes is generally a lifestyle condition that can be prevented.
- A combined therapy of medication, rest, low-impact aerobic exercise, and physical therapy can manage most types of chronic pain.
- Many conditions associated with chronic pain have a genetic component.

Pain Management in Children

In This Chapter

- Earaches, sore throats, and stomach pain
- Injuries and trauma
- Diseases and syndromes causing pain
- Early detection and pain management

Headaches, abdominal pain, and fractures are the most common pain complaints in children, and diagnosing the reason for pain in young children can be difficult. Pediatric medicine is a specialty practice for good reasons, as diagnosis and treatment for children present unique challenges. In addition to the usual bumps and scrapes of childhood, certain infections and medical conditions can cause pain. In this chapter, you'll learn about many causes of pain in children and how they're treated.

When to See the Doctor

Things happen quickly with children, and many painful conditions, such as injuries and illnesses common to children, are difficult to foresee and prevent. A simple fever can be a sign of a serious illness, but severe abdominal cramping may not be anything more than gas pains. Waiting to see what happens is not the best course of action, however, and sometimes just a phone call to your child's doctor will give you reassurance and the necessary information to help your child get better quickly.

The bottom line: Use the 24-hour rule. After 24 hours, if your child has been uncomfortable, is in pain, or you can tell that he isn't feeling well, call your doctor. She's there to answer your questions, put your mind at ease, and oversee your child's health. If the problem is severe, don't wait that long. An hour in pain can feel like a week.

Diagnosis

Pediatricians are skilled diagnosticians, and this is important since their youngest patients cannot tell the doctor where they are hurting. Your child's doctor will listen to your account of symptoms and then conduct a thorough physical examination of your child. In many cases, tissue cultures are needed to determine the source of a bacterial infection. These cultures may be taken from the nose, throat, urine, or stool.

Ear Infections

Cold season can start with the beginning of the school year and continue until summer, or so it seems, and that season can go year round if your child goes to daycare or is around other children every day. Colds are so common that we tend to associate childhood with runny noses, but sometimes these runny and stuffy noses, sniffles, and sneezes turn into ear infections, and these infections hurt.

 SPEAKING OF PAIN

Breastfeeding has been found to lower the incidence of ear infections in children.

You may have heard an ear infection referred to as a "cold in the ear," but that's a rather vague description of what's going on. The medical term is acute otitis media, and it simply means acute infection of the middle ear.

Parts of the Ear

The ear is divided into three sections: outer, middle, and inner. The outer ear is the part you can see. The opening in the outer ear leads to the external ear canal, and that goes to the eardrum.

The middle ear is made up of the eardrum and a cavity on the other side of the eardrum. From this cavity, a tube, called the Eustachian tube, leads to the pharynx. Three small bones here connect the eardrum to the inner ear. This is the part that's frequently the site of ear infections.

The inner ear is the most complicated of the three parts. It contains nerves, passageways, and cavities, all with specialized functions that transmit sound.

Causes of Ear Infection

The Eustachian tubes are designed to let fluid drain from the middle ear. In children, these tubes are much shorter than those of adults, so when your child has a cold, it doesn't take much to block them. The virus can infect the Eustachian tubes, causing them to swell up and get blocked with thick mucus. A bacterial infection can have the same results. Childhood allergies can also cause the Eustachian tubes to swell and become blocked.

Whether viral or bacterial, this mucus then becomes a breeding ground for bacteria, building up pressure in the tubes and causing pain. In many cases these infections clear up within a week or two, but sometimes they go on longer and become chronic.

Ear infections are very common in children, with many identified risk factors. Having had one ear infection increases your child's risk of contracting another. There may also be a genetic connection, since these tend to run in families. Boys tend to be more susceptible to them than girls. Other risk factors include the following:

- Exposure to secondhand smoke
- Having had low birth weight or having been born prematurely
- Using a pacifier or going to bed with a bottle

Symptoms of an ear infection are pain and fever. Your child may try to put a finger in her ear or tug at her ear. Young children may cry, and older ones too, for that matter, because ear infections are very painful. Your child may not feel like playing or even eating, and she may not hear what you are saying.

You can give your child nonaspirin nonsteroidal anti-inflammatory drugs (NSAIDs), such as Children's Tylenol, Children's Motrin, or Children's Advil, to help relieve the pain.

Once at the doctor's office, your pediatrician will conduct a physical examination that includes looking into your child's ear with an instrument called an *otoscope*. She may take a cotton swab and take a sample of the mucus to send to the lab for testing to see whether the infection is caused by a bacteria.

DEFINITION

An **otoscope** is a handheld device with a light and a funnel-shaped attachment at one end. The attachment fits into the external ear canal, and the light allows the doctor to see inside the ear.

Bacterial infections can be treated with antibiotics, but antibiotics aren't effective against viruses. If a virus is suspected, the doctor may prescribe ear drops and a pain reliever, such as the ones indicated previously.

A heating pad set on the lowest setting and wrapped in a protective cover, such as a towel, can be held against your child's ear to give comfort.

If your child has repeated bouts of ear infections or if the current infection is persisting beyond three months, your physician may recommend surgery to place tubes in the eardrums. These tubes allow the fluid to drain and air to enter, so that the pressure in the Eustachian tubes doesn't build up. Your child will need a general anesthetic for this procedure, which is usually done on an outpatient basis.

The tubes remain in the eardrum until they fall out on their own. This takes about a year. In some cases, when they don't fall out, they'll need to be removed by the physician. While your child has tubes, it's important to keep water from entering the ears, so earplugs can be helpful when bathing or swimming. Fortunately, most children outgrow ear infections.

Tonsillitis

Your tonsils, those tissue clumps at the back of your throat, are part of your body's immune defense system. Sometimes, however, they get overwhelmed and aren't capable of preventing illness. In these cases, instead of protecting the body they incubate bacteria and viruses, become inflamed, and can hurt. A sore throat can feel like anything from a mild scratch to an excruciating stab.

When is a sore throat just a minor discomfort, and when is it something more serious? It can be difficult to tell. Sore throats are common in children, and most of the time they're just an annoying accompaniment to the common cold. Sometimes, however, more is involved than just a scratchy throat.

Tonsillitis means inflammation of the tonsils and is usually caused by a virus or a bacteria. Most children experience tonsillitis at least once, and for some it's a recurring problem. Symptoms and treatment vary, based on what kind of tonsillitis your child has.

In acute tonsillitis, the symptoms come on quickly, last a few days, and then resolve over the course of a week or so. In addition to a sore throat, your child may have a fever and feel ill. Swallowing is difficult because of the pain and the lymph nodes in the neck are usually swollen. Your child's breath will smell very bad because of the infection. In chronic tonsillitis, your child's throat seems to perpetually hurt, the lymph nodes are always swollen, and she has persistent bad breath.

A more serious sore throat is strep throat, caused by a bacteria, *A. streptococcus.* Symptoms of strep throat include white and red spots on the tonsils, abdominal pain, a rash, and headache.

Diagnosis is made based upon symptoms, a physical examination, and a throat culture. For a throat culture, the doctor takes a cotton swab and wipes the tissues in the back of the mouth to collect a sample of the bacteria. He then wipes the sample onto a special culture-growing medium and allows it to grow. If it is streptococcus, results will be positive in two days.

Unfortunately, having a throat culture done isn't a comfortable procedure. It doesn't hurt, but the throat is already sore, and having anything inserted in the mouth doesn't feel good. The doctor may need to use a tongue depressor to keep the tongue from fighting the swab, and your child may gag as the swab is wiped over the tonsils.

POINTERS ON PAIN

If your child is young, holding him on your lap while the procedure is done may help. An older child can help by holding the tongue depressor. In any regard, the swab takes only a few seconds.

While waiting for the results, if your physician suspects that strep is present, she may begin your child on a course of antibiotics. It's important to finish the prescribed course of medication so the symptoms don't return.

For viral sore throats, rest, a children's nonaspirin pain reliever, and plenty of fluids to prevent dehydration are recommended.

If your child has chronic tonsillitis, your pediatrician may recommend a tonsillectomy, which is the surgical removal of the tonsils. Tonsillectomies used to be a routine childhood medical procedure. Today, due to improved antibiotics, they're not as routine, but if chronic tonsillitis is making your child miserable, it's often the best option.

Headaches

Headaches may seem more like an adult affliction than one affecting children, but it's estimated that at least 40 percent of children experience a headache before they're seven years old. By the time they're 15, 75 percent have had at least one headache.

Most of the time children have headaches for the same reasons adults do: the flu, stress, or tension. Children are subject to many of the same stressors as adults. Migraines can also begin in childhood, and they often occur at surprisingly early ages—sometimes in children as young as 5. If migraines tend to run in your family, it's important to share this information with your pediatrician, as it can help in both diagnosis and treatment.

If your child doesn't have a head cold or the flu, a headache may be a symptom of a more serious medical condition. If a headache comes on after a fall, this could be potentially serious as well. Always check with your doctor to rule out the possibility of an underlying medical condition as the source of the headache.

Diagnosis of the cause may include blood tests, x-rays, CT scan, or an MRI. Treatment may include rest, prescription or over-the-counter medications, changes in diet, and increased exercise. Play is an excellent outlet for stress in children.

Abdominal Pain

It's difficult for a parent or caregiver to determine whether pain in the abdomen is serious or not. Gas, constipation, infection, food poisoning, and numerous other possibilities make abdominal pain a very common reason for taking a child to the doctor.

POINTERS ON PAIN

Trust your instincts as a parent. You know when your child is hurting, and you shouldn't be concerned at all about "bothering the doctor."

If your child has had abdominal pain for more than one day, check in with the doctor. Most acute pain is gone by then. If your child has a pre-existing medical condition such as sickle cell anemia or diabetes, or if you suspect poisoning or another serious problem, don't wait at all.

Often abdominal pain comes with other symptoms, such as vomiting, diarrhea, or fever. Many times abdominal pain is the result of a bacterial or viral infection, and children who are sick generally look sick. This can help differentiate the pain associated with colic or constipation from a more serious cause.

Diagnosis is made based upon symptoms and a medical examination. Tell the doctor what you have done to provide treatment for your child—for example, if you've given any pain relievers, tried any home remedies, or used any herbal preparations.

During the examination, the doctor will press on different parts of the abdomen to see whether any particular place is more painful than others. Blood, urine, and stool samples will be sent to the lab for analysis. Diagnostic imaging tests, such as ultrasound, may be indicated.

Depending upon the results of the physical examination and while awaiting the results of the lab tests, the doctor will either send you and your child home or admit your child to the hospital for observation and possible surgery.

If you're sent home, you'll be given a written set of instructions advising you on how to care for your child to help speed recovery. Generally these include rest, a special diet of soft, bland foods (mashed bananas are a favorite), and liquids (such as ginger ale or broths) to prevent dehydration. Infants are often prescribed Pedialyte, which can be obtained over the counter at drugstores or major grocery stores.

STABS AND JABS

Milk and carbonated beverages can aggravate symptoms of diarrhea, so avoid these until your child is feeling better. Also, power drinks such as Gatorade aren't recommended because their sugar content is too high for young children.

When your child is feeling better, reintroduce solid foods gradually. Just as children can get sick quickly, they can bounce back quickly. In most cases, your child will let you know, either in words or actions, when she's feeling back to par.

Scoliosis

The normal spine appears straight up and down when viewed from the back. In scoliosis, however, the spine curves to the left or to the right, and sometimes more than one curve is present. If the curve(s) are extreme, they put unnatural pressure on different parts of the spine, causing deformity and problems later on. According to the National Institutes of Health, three to five children per thousand have spinal curves that are considered severe enough to require treatment.

The most common type of scoliosis is adolescent idiopathic scoliosis, a term that means the cause isn't known. Girls are more likely than boys to have scoliosis, and there seems to be a genetic component to this condition, as it tends to run in families.

Scoliosis is usually diagnosed during a routine physical examination, and many schools conduct annual scoliosis screenings. If the curve seems severe, your physician may recommend x-rays to determine the extent of the curvature. Using the x-rays as a guide, measurements of the curves are taken, and any curves in excess of 20 degrees are candidates for treatment.

Treatment options include expectant management, bracing, or surgery.

Growing Pains

You've undoubtedly heard this term before. It refers to the achy pain children get in their legs and, although it doesn't have anything specifically to do with growing, it does seem to be related to the demands children place on their developing musculo-skeletal systems. It's estimated that about 20 percent of children between the ages of 2 and 12 experience growing pains, which tend to stop when puberty begins. Girls seem to be bothered with growing pains more than boys. Some believe that growing pains causing leg pain are from shin splints or flat feet. Children often run more than adults and don't wear shoes. Both could contribute to the leg pains.

Growing pains symptoms follow a typical pattern. Often, your child may wake up in the middle of the night complaining that her legs hurt. You may fear the worst, but no fever or any signs of inflammation are present. You try a gentle massaging of the legs, which seems to help, and your child falls asleep again. In the morning, the legs are free from pain. It's puzzling and troublesome.

Diagnosis is usually made based upon symptoms, and a physical examination can rule out other causes for your child's discomfort. There's no specific treatment indicated for growing pains, but gentle leg massage can be comforting, along with a heating pad. You can try Children's Tylenol or another children's pain reliever, if the pain is too troublesome.

Osgood-Schlatter Disease

Osgood-Schlatter disease is found usually in physically active children and adolescents. Many young athletes experience this condition, which can cause pain below the knee at the place where the shinbone connects to the kneecap. As the tendon becomes stressed, a painful lump forms. Activity causes the pain to get worse, and the thigh muscles may feel tight.

 SPEAKING OF PAIN

It's estimated that around 20 percent of active adolescent athletes experience Osgood-Schlatter disease.

It may be that abnormal stresses placed on growing joints are responsible, as the symptoms generally resolve after the major growth spurts have ended.

Diagnosis is made based upon symptoms, medical history, and a physical examination. Diagnostic imaging tests, such as x-rays, may be recommended to confirm the diagnosis.

Treatment involves use of NSAIDs, rest, icing, and proper stretching warm-ups and cool-downs after physical activity. Proper coaching techniques for supervising young athletes is an area of concern here. Be sure your child is wearing protective gear, including knee pads. In some cases, physical therapy may be recommended to help stretch the tendon properly.

Nursemaid's Elbow

Nursemaid's elbow isn't a condition that affects caregivers of children, even though the name may lead you to think this is the case. It's actually something that caregivers do that causes this condition in children.

Have you ever taken your child's hands and twirled her around? Or have you ever walked with your spouse or partner with a child between you, each one of you holding a child's hand and then swinging him up to the curb? It's something we all do, and it's a prime cause of nursemaid's elbow, which simply is a partial dislocation of the elbow joint.

The medical term for nursemaid's elbow is radial head dislocation. Symptoms begin immediately, and the child will cry and not want the affected arm touched. She may hold her arm against her stomach to keep it still. The acute pain can go away, but the child still won't bend the arm at the elbow. To the naked eye, the arm doesn't appear to be deformed. This is because it's a partial dislocation.

The problem occurs because a young child's joints aren't strong enough to handle extreme stress. Unfortunately, if the elbow has dislocated once, it's more likely to dislocate again. Nursemaid's elbow doesn't usually affect children over the age of 5.

Nursemaid's elbow requires immediate medical assistance. Do not try to straighten the arm. You can apply a splint to the arm, but don't change its position while you're doing so. An ice pack can help relieve the pain while you're en route to the emergency room or doctor's office.

The doctor will gently manipulate the elbow back into proper position. With prompt treatment, there are usually no lasting ill effects.

You can prevent nursemaid's elbow and still enjoy playing with your child. The fix is simple: lift your child from under the arms and not by the hands or wrists.

Ehler Danlos Syndrome

Ehler Danlos syndrome is a genetically transmitted group of conditions with certain common features. These features include loose joints (hypermobility); generalized tissue weakness; and skin that bruises, tears, and stretches easily.

Because of the looseness of the joints, dislocations are frequent, and scoliosis (curvature of the spine) is a common complication. In one form of this syndrome, the arteries and bowel may rupture without warning.

Diagnosis is made based upon evaluation of symptoms, a physical examination, and a skin biopsy and tissue culture to discover both the presence of the syndrome along with its specific form.

Prevention of injury to the skin and joints is of critical importance. Use sunscreen and wear protective clothing to guard against sunburns and minor injuries, such as cuts and scrapes, which can be difficult to treat. Since the skin is so fragile, suturing cuts can pose serious problems.

POINTERS ON PAIN

Parenting a child with a serious medical condition is difficult. Contact the Ehlers Danlos Support Group at www.ehlers-danlos.org.

Exercise is recommended to help strengthen the muscles and increase their ability to stabilize the joints. Your physician may refer you to a physical therapist for help in developing an appropriate exercise program for your child. An occupational therapist can help with designing and fashioning braces to protect your child's joints.

Marfan's Syndrome

Marfan's syndrome is a genetically transmitted disorder that affects the body's connective tissues. It occurs when a gene mutates, or changes, and in this case, it affects the gene responsible for producing a protein essential to the health of connective tissue. This protein is called fibrillin.

POINTERS ON PAIN

Scoliosis is common in children with Marfan's syndrome. Bracing may be needed to provide stability to the spine.

Fibrillin is what gives the body's tissues their resilience, so that when they stretch they have the capability of returning to their original shape and size. Without fibrillin, there's no support, and this lack of support has far-reaching effects throughout the body.

Symptoms involve the musculoskeletal system, cardiovascular system, and eyes. The outward appearance of someone with Marfan's syndrome is an important diagnostic clue. It seems that almost everything about a child with Marfan's is long and slender and loose.

Marfan's syndrome cannot be cured, but the various symptoms of leg, back, and abdominal pain can be treated.

STABS AND JABS

Prevention of infection is an important concern for children with Marfan's. If your child will be having dental work or surgery, your physician may prescribe a course of antibiotics prior to the procedure.

Yearly eye examinations are essential, and eye problems should be treated aggressively to prevent loss of vision. During this exam, the opthalmologist will measure eye pressure to check for early signs of glaucoma. If necessary, she will prescribe eye drops to reduce this pressure. In some cases, surgery may be indicated.

If the lens is dislocated, your ophthalmologist may prescribe daily eye drops and corrective glasses. In some cases, surgery may be necessary. Cataracts can be removed surgically.

STABS AND JABS

A retinal detachment is a medical emergency. If your child says she is seeing flashes of light or if her vision suddenly blurs, seek immediate medical assistance to prevent permanent loss of vision.

The sooner your child is diagnosed, the sooner treatment for symptoms can begin. Today, many children with Marfan's can look forward to a normal life span.

Legg Calve Perthes Syndrome

Legg Calve Perthes syndrome affects the hip joint, and more specifically the tip of the femur (thigh bone) that inserts into the hip socket. For some reason that doctors don't understand, sometimes blood flow to the end of the bone is decreased, causing the bone to die. The dead bone separates from the healthy bone, causing the rounded ball end of the femur to flatten out.

This condition is more common in young boys between the ages of 4 and 10 and usually affects just one hip. Over the next two to three years, blood supply is restored, new bone cells grow, and the bone reforms. The earliest symptom is a limp, although the child may not complain of pain.

Later symptoms include pain in the knee, thigh, or groin. The muscles may atrophy in the upper thigh of the joint that's affected, and the leg may not grow at the same rate as the nonaffected leg. Range of motion of the affected leg also decreases, and it becomes noticeably stiff.

Diagnosis is made based upon evaluation of symptoms and a physical examination that includes x-rays of the thigh and hip area.

Treatment is focused on keeping the end of the femur inside the socket. Your doctor may prescribe nonsteroidal anti-inflammatory children's medications and physical therapy to restore range of motion and strengthen the muscles supporting the joint. Sometimes a brace is recommended to keep the joint stable. In some cases surgery may be indicated to repair the joint.

The outlook to a large degree depends upon how old your child is when the condition develops. The younger the child, the more encouraging the outcome. Children over

6 years of age may have some permanent hip deformity, even with treatment, and osteoarthritis is likely to develop in that joint later.

Prevention

Teach your child to wash hands after play and after using the bathroom. Practicing good hygiene can go a long way toward preventing childhood illnesses. If you have a family history of a genetically caused illness, such as Marfan's syndrome or Ehler Danlos syndrome, genetic counseling before pregnancy is a wise decision.

Treatment

Treatment for pain issues in children centers around treating the condition that's causing the pain. Pain is not an illness—it's a symptom—and the potential reasons why a child is feeling pain are almost limitless.

As a parent, trust your instincts. You know when your child is hurting, and you know when that hurt is the sign of a bigger problem than a simple stubbed toe or colic pain. You will never regret getting medical advice for your child's symptoms, and help is as close as your telephone.

The Least You Need to Know

- The severity of pain in children isn't a good indicator of the seriousness of the problem. Always check with your doctor when you have concerns.
- Earaches are a common problem with children, but recurring earaches or an infection lasting more than three months may require surgical intervention.
- A strep throat infection requires antibiotics for treatment.
- Abdominal pain lasting more than a day should be evaluated by your child's pediatrician.
- Young athletes need proper warm-ups and cool-downs to prevent joint injuries.
- Trust your instincts when your child has pain. If you suspect there's a problem, there probably is.

Hope for the Future

In This Chapter

- Funding for research
- Joining a national organization
- Considering a clinical trial
- Advocating for your future

Pain has been present since the beginning of time, and if you're suffering, you may wonder why science hasn't been able to eliminate it once and for all. Pain is multifactorial, which means that pain is complex in nature. So the cure for one type of pain may not have any effect on a different type. This chapter takes a look ahead at what's on the horizon as scientists work to make the goal of eradicating chronic pain a reality.

Pain is limiting. It wraps a tight border around your world and does its best to keep you inside its boundaries. Fortunately, pain has limits as well. It's not all-powerful, and it can be conquered. The researchers working to end chronic pain refuse to accept pain's limitations, and so they ask a simple question: "What if?" These two words form the base upon which all research is constructed.

Pain Research Studies

Pain is the number-one reason people visit their physicians. It's responsible for lost work days, loss of productivity while on the job, and decreased enjoyment of recreational activities outside the workplace. The problem is receiving national attention. In 2000, the U.S. Congress passed a provision, signed by the president, that declared that the decade beginning January 1, 2001, would be the Decade of Pain Control and Research.

When we feel pain, we focus on the what and the where, but researchers look at the why and the how. A diverse group of individuals and agencies fund research, which is an incredibly expensive undertaking.

One of the primary funding agencies is the National Institutes of Health (NIH), a service of the U.S. Department of Health and Human Services. NIH supports biomedical research and clinical trials and is your best first stop for education. The website for the NIH is http://clinicalresearch.nih.gov/index.html.

Exciting research is taking off in all directions at NIH. Current projects include studying how to synthesize the body's natural painkillers and make them available as medications for treating pain. These naturally occurring substances, such as serotonin, norepinephrine, and opioidlike chemicals, are found in the spinal cord. Additionally, scientists are looking into the role that peptides play in pain response. Peptides are compounds that make up proteins. Current research is examining the role of such peptides to treat varying degrees of pain.

The search for pain relief is leading researchers in some promising directions, as they look for strong pain relievers that don't come with downsides. One study is examining how snail venom may provide some interesting results for managing pain. Other research is studying the pain-relieving potential of suboxone (buphennorphine), currently used to treat opioid dependence.

POINTERS ON PAIN

Eliminating all pain is not science's goal. The acute pain response is essential to survival. The object of research is to find a way to help manage both acute and chronic pain better.

Other research is studying the link between the immune system and the nervous system. The link in question is a type of protein called cytokine. Cytokines promote inflammation that sets off the pain response, even if there's no injury involved. The goal of this research is to develop a new class of pain medications targeted at controlling cytokine levels.

In the brain, glia cells are also a focus of research. These cells make up over 70 percent of the cells in the brain and spinal cord. Their job is as first responders when there's injury to the central nervous system (CNS). Once researchers have discovered the exact mechanism that activates these cells, they may be able to regulate their release. That discovery may mean big gains in pain relief.

To read more exciting news about what's going on with research into pain, visit the NIH website.

National Organizations

Most medical conditions have a national organization, devoted to advocacy, research, and dissemination of information. Most of these are volunteer and nonprofit or not-for-profit groups. Your physician can give you the name of the national organization appropriate to your condition.

The Arthritis Foundation

The Arthritis Foundation (www.arthritis.org) provides funding opportunities and research updates and supports advocacy for the 46 million Americans living with arthritis.

SPEAKING OF PAIN

Since 1948, The Arthritis Foundation has contributed approximately $400 million to research and annually funds 200 to 300 researchers in 100 institutions nationwide.

Predictions by the Arthritis Foundation for the next 10 to 25 years, given adequate funding, include the following:

- Identification of the specific genes associated with different types of arthritis, leading to genetic testing and therapy

- Use of biomarkers and imaging tests to diagnose arthritis before the onset of symptoms

- Vaccines to prevent some forms of arthritis

- Joint reconstruction and tissue engineering to resurface worn joints and replace worn cartilage

Research has already begun on turning these goals into a reality. Significant progress is being made on studies of the immune system's role and in identification of genetic factors that may lead to the onset of arthritis symptoms.

The American Fibromyalgia Syndrome Association

This nonprofit, all-volunteer organization solicits donations to fund research into the causes and treatments for fibromyalgia. About 90 percent of donations go directly to fund research.

Current research projects are studying abnormalities in the CNS believed to be responsible for many symptoms of fibromyalgia: widespread muscular pain, sleep and digestive disorders, chronic headaches, memory and concentration difficulties, and other symptoms. Current funded research is studying myofascial trigger points, use of low-dose Naltrexone to treat fibromyalgia, and the impact of fibromyalgia on brain aging and cognitive function. The association's website is www.afsafund.org.

The American Cancer Society

The American Cancer Society targets both research and advocacy programs. It is the nation's largest private, not-for-profit source for funds for cancer research. Since it began in 1946, it has committed about $3.4 billion to cancer research.

The *human genome project* continues to provide cancer researchers with abundant resources for their investigations. One area of research is focusing on a system's approach to cancer—studying how multiple events at the molecular level can trigger the development of cancer cells. This is a radical shift from the single gene or protein approach.

DEFINITION

The **human genome project** was a scientific endeavor completed in 2003 that resulted in sequencing and mapping every gene in the human body.

Current research into prostate cancer has identified four different markers that, when present together, may lead to a urine test with the capability of predicting prostate cancer. Early detection holds the best chance of a positive outcome, and these signature markers may eventually lead to a cure.

Other research continues, and cancer, once a death sentence, is moving into the arena of chronically manageable diseases, the next step on the way to the cure for all cancers. The American Cancer Society's website is www.cancer.org.

The American Heart Association

The American Heart Association is a national volunteer health organization, founded in 1924 with a mission to share research findings and promote study into heart disease. Its goal is to reduce coronary artery disease, stroke, and risk by 25 percent by 2010.

You can find information on the prevention of heart disease and stroke on their website, along with additional information on cardiovascular health. Their website is www.americanheart.org.

The American Diabetes Association

The American Diabetes Association partners with the National Institutes of Health to conduct research into diabetes. Recent studies have looked into treatments for diabetic retinopathy, a common complication of diabetes that can result in blindness in both type 1 and type 2 diabetes.

STABS AND JABS

New research in diabetes is focusing on how obesity contributes to cardiovascular risks in type 2 diabetes. Such research underscores the importance of maintaining a proper weight if you are diabetic.

One promising study is looking into how restoring leptin sensitivity in the brain can help return insulin levels to normal. The association's website is www.diabetes.org.

Clinical Trials

Once the research discoveries have been made, the next step is testing them to see whether they hold promise in treating the various medical conditions that cause pain. The National Institutes of Health sponsors a plethora of clinical trials, and if you're interested in participating, this is the place to start. You can find a complete listing of available clinical trials along with instructions for joining them at the NIH website: http://ClinicalTrials.gov.

The NIH reports that ClinicalTrials.gov currently contains 81,152 trials sponsored by the National Institutes of Health, other federal agencies, and private industry. Studies listed in the database are conducted in all 50 states and in 170 countries.

There are various kinds of clinical trials, and each trial consists of specific phases. The NIH offers the following information about types of clinical trials:

- **Treatment trials**—These test new approaches to surgery or radiation therapy, new combinations of drugs, or new treatments.

- **Prevention trials**—These look for better means of preventing disease from occurring in people who have not had the particular disease or for a way to prevent the disease from recurring in those who have previously had it.

- **Diagnostic trials**—These trials determine better diagnostic procedures for detecting disease or a particular medical condition.

- **Screening trials**—Screening trials test the best way to detect certain diseases or health conditions.

- **Quality of life trials**—Also known as supportive care trials, these explore and measure ways to improve comfort and quality of life for people with chronic illness.

Deciding to join a clinical trial requires a commitment. You agree to participate for the duration of the trial and to follow the protocol of that trial. (The protocol is the method by which the trial will be conducted.) You may leave a trial at any time, but if you do, valuable information will be lost. Before you make the decision to participate, weigh the pros and cons carefully.

The Upside of Participating in a Clinical Trial

Besides the altruistic aspects of contributing to the public good, the benefits to you include access to new drugs, procedures, or therapy before they're available to the general public. You'll also have enhanced access to personal medical care while you're a participant. Living with pain can make you feel a loss of control over your body. Participating in a clinical trial can empower you and help you manage pain more effectively.

The Downside of Participating in a Clinical Trial

There are no guarantees that the drug, procedure, or treatment therapy will be effective. The side effects or complications of an experimental treatment aren't completely known yet, so you risk severe, potentially life-altering side effects. That's the risk you take when you sign on. It's important to go into this venture with hopeful but reasonable expectations.

Another downside is that even if the trial is a success, you could be among the group who received the *placebo*, meaning you'll have to wait for the results of the trial to be evaluated and the drug, procedure, or treatment to be made available to the public before you can benefit. One interesting phenomenon in scientific research is known as the placebo effect, and it shows how powerful the mind-body connection is. In some cases, people receiving the placebo have experienced improvement, sometimes significant improvement, in their symptoms. Because the mind believes the substance is working, it does.

DEFINITION

A **placebo** is a harmless substance or procedure that is used with a control group in a medical study. The placebo does not contain the substance or use the procedure being tested. It's used to evaluate the effects of a treatment in a comparison study.

A commitment of your time must be made as well. You may be required to check in with the research team frequently during the trial, and this may become inconvenient. The final decision is yours.

Meeting the Criteria

After you've made the decision to participate in a clinical trial, your application will be evaluated to see whether you meet the criteria established for that trial. These guidelines are essential to the success of the trial. Each clinical trial is different, and each one will have different inclusion (you meet the criteria) or exclusion (you don't meet the criteria) guidelines. Some common criteria used to evaluate you include the following:

- Age
- Gender
- Type and stage of your medical condition
- Previous medications used to treat the condition

Depending upon the specific trial, there may be other criteria as well.

STABS AND JABS

If you're not chosen for a clinical trial, it's not a reflection of your moral character. It's simply a matter of not being the right fit for that particular trial.

Informed Consent

Congratulations! You've been accepted to participate in the trial. Now what? The next step involves giving informed consent. The trial has selected you; now it's your turn to evaluate the trial and decide whether you want to continue with it.

Informed consent means you understand any potential risks that may occur with the trial, and you agree to abide by the conditions and protocol of the trial. You also agree that you will stay with the study until its conclusion. The informed consent document will lay out the specific details of the study, including how long it will last and what will be expected of you.

Even if you sign the consent form, you are still free to leave the study at any time. It is important to inform the study personnel if you must leave the study and explain your reasons for leaving. This gives them valuable information, even if your continued participation isn't possible.

Although many of the following questions are covered in the informed consent form, the National Institutes of Health recommend you ask the following questions before you commit to a clinical trial:

1. What is the purpose of the study?

2. Who is going to be in the study?

3. Why do researchers believe the experimental treatment being tested may be effective? Has it been tested before?

4. What kinds of tests and experimental treatments are involved?

5. How do the possible risks, side effects, and benefits in the study compare with my current treatment?

6. How might this trial affect my daily life?

7. How long will the trial last?

8. Will hospitalization be required?

9. Who will pay for the experimental treatment?

10. Will I be reimbursed for other expenses?

11. What type of long-term follow-up care is part of this study?

12. How will I know that the experimental treatment is working? Will results of the trials be provided to me?

13. Who will be in charge of my care?

The answers to these questions will help you make an informed decision about whether or not to participate. Either write down the answers or take along a portable tape recorder so you'll have the information on file.

The Study Team

Clinical trials are conducted in many settings, which can include your doctor's office, local hospital, clinic, or university. In addition to you (a very important team member) and other study participants, other team members will include doctors, nurses, social workers, and researchers. You'll most likely have a physical examination at the beginning of the trial as well as at key points along the duration of the trial.

If you have any questions, the team will answer most of them. You'll be told whether a placebo is being used in the trial, although you most likely won't be told if you're in the control group (getting the placebo) or in the group that's receiving the drug, procedure, or other therapy. If receiving the placebo would interfere with your current treatment therapy or would place your health at risk, you would not be included in the control group unless this information was divulged to you prior to commencement of the study. If you might be harmed by the procedure, you might be excluded from the study on these grounds.

POINTERS ON PAIN

According to federal regulations, your privacy while participating in a clinical trial is assured. Your real name or any identifying characteristics cannot be used in any published data concerning the trial.

During the study, you'll continue with your own primary health-care physician, pain medicine specialist, or other specialty practice physician. Notify your own doctors of your participation in the study so that they will be able to monitor your health during the trial.

Safeguards

In addition to the informed consent agreement, you have additional backup to ensure that you will be exposed to the least possible risk and that the clinical trial is justified, based upon expected outcomes. The entity that oversees this responsibility is an Institutional Review Board (IRB). Every clinical trial conducted in the United States is approved and monitored by one of these IRBs.

The IRB is made up of an independent group of physicians, statisticians, and community advocates. In addition to granting permission for the study to begin, the IRB continues to monitor the study throughout its life span. This monitoring is important because many sponsoring entities of clinical trials have a vested interest in the outcome. For example, in addition to federal agencies, pharmaceutical companies sponsor clinical trials.

Phases of Clinical Trials

Clinical trials have four phases. Each phase is designed to address a specific issue concerning the drug, procedure, or treatment under study. The NIH lists these phases as follows:

- **Phase I**—The first test of the experimental drug, procedure, or treatment on a small group of people (20 to 80) to evaluate overall safety, calculate a safe dosage range, and look for side effects.

- **Phase II**—The experimental drug, procedure, or treatment is now administered to a larger group of people (100 to 300) to continue the evaluative process.

- **Phase III**—The experimental drug, procedure, or treatment is now given to a much larger population (1,000 to 3,000). In this phase, researchers are comparing it to currently available treatments and evaluating its safety and efficacy.

- **Phase IV**—The experimental drug, procedure, or treatment is now on the market. Researchers are fine-tuning information on risks, benefits, and optimal use.

These phases are conducted over an extended time span of several years, so you most likely will not be involved in every phase of the study. It's common to be part of just one phase. It takes years for a drug to be approved by the Food and Drug

Administration. The process is expensive, as well as lengthy. It takes at least five to eight years for a new drug to go from inception to marketing, and each one is estimated to cost more than $800 million.

Being part of the research process not only will give you an appreciation for the process, it will also give you an opportunity to become an advocate for pain relief in the area of your own medical condition.

The Importance of Advocacy

Each year legislators introduce various bills into Congress for funding for various medical conditions. Without public support, many of these bills die in the House of Representatives. It is important to support the national organization that's advocating for you. Whether you have arthritis, heart disease, diabetes, or any medical condition that has pain as a symptom, a national organization is fighting for you.

Join the local, regional, or national chapter of your association and let your voice be heard. Keep informed by consulting their websites, and when legislation is pending, use the forms many of them provide to let your legislators know you support funding for research. Congress is spending your tax dollars, so speak up and support funding for medical research to be sure you're getting a good return on your investment.

Numerous advocacy groups are working to advance the cause of medical research. The Research Advocacy Network (RAN) is one of these groups. A nonprofit organization, RAN's mission is "to bring together all participants in the medical research process with the focus on education, support, and connecting patient advocates with the research community to improve patient care." Their website is http://researchadvocacy.org.

RAN reports that there are currently 395 cancer treatments in some phase of clinical trials, but just 5 percent of the adult population currently is participating in trials. Increasing public involvement in advocacy and in participating in clinical trials will help speed the process.

The outlook is good for a day when chronic pain will be just a distant echo from the past. Each day another researcher asks the question, "What if?" And the investigative process begins anew. Research will give us the answers to the mysteries of pain. Each day, the work continues. Support research, become an advocate, and be a part of this promising future.

The Least You Need to Know

- The National Institutes of Health (NIH) is the nation's largest supporter of medical research.
- Each medical condition most likely has a national organization that provides information, advocacy, and research support.
- Joining a clinical trial can give you early access to new drugs, treatments, and procedures.
- Advocacy is the way to let your voice be heard when Congress considers funding for medical research.

Glossary

active rest   Balanced program of rest and mild low-impact aerobic exercise.

affirmations   Positive self-talk. They're designed to increase your self-esteem, promote a sense of well-being, and give you control over negative situations.

amitriptyline   Medication used to treat depression. Marketed under the names Elavil and Endep.

analgesic   Drug used for pain relief that may or may not have anti-inflammatory properties. It works by blocking pain receptors in the central nervous system.

anemia   A low red blood cell count.

aneurysm   An abnormal, localized widening of a blood vessel. This results in a bulge that weakens the wall of the blood vessel. An aneurysm can burst at any time and is life-threatening.

ankylosing spondylitis   Type of inflammatory arthritis affecting the joints and ligaments of the spine.

anticonvulsants   Class of medications used to treat seizure disorders that have been found to have some benefit in treating symptoms of migraine.

antidepressants   Class of medications used to treat depression that have been found to have some benefit in treating symptoms of migraine.

arthrocentesis   Medical procedure used to collect fluid from a joint by means of a syringe.

autoimmune disease   Condition in which the body's immune system malfunctions and decides that the body is an invader, instead of the entity it is supposed to protect. In the case of rheumatoid arthritis, the immune system targets the joint lining, eventually destroying it.

biologics   Also referred to as biologic response modifiers (BRMs). Newer class of disease-modifying antirheumatic drugs that target specific parts of the immune system. Often used to treat symptoms of rheumatoid arthritis, ankylosing spondylitis, psoriatic arthritis, and other rheumatologic conditions. *See also* disease-modifying antirheumatic drugs (DMARDs).

bursa   Sac filled with lubricating fluid, located between tissues of the body or at pressure points such as the elbow.

bursitis   Inflammation of the bursa.

capsaicin   Substance found in different kinds of hot peppers, responsible for making them "hot."

carpal tunnel   Bony structure in the wrist that houses the carpal nerve.

catheter   Flexible, hollow tube that can be inserted in a venous structure or body cavity to deliver medication or fluids, widen a narrowed passageway, or remove body fluids for analysis.

cholecystectomy   Surgical removal of the gallbladder.

colonoscopy   Procedure in which the physician inserts a flexible tube equipped with a camera into the rectum and up into the colon to look for abnormalities. The pictures are transmitted to a computer screen in real time.

complex regional pain syndrome   Also referred to as central pain syndrome. Condition referring to pain resulting from damage to the central nervous system.

compression fracture   Occurs when the vertebrae of the spine are first subjected to severe jarring and then come crashing together. If the force of the impact is hard enough, the bones break.

coronary artery disease (CAD)   Refers to damage to arteries that supply the heart with blood, nutrients, and oxygen. Often caused by plaque buildup within the arteries.

corticosteroid   *See* steroids.

crystalline arthritis   Type of arthritis in which deposits of uric acid or calcium phyrophosphate crystals are deposited in joints of the body.

cyclosporine   Medication used to treat rheumatoid arthritis.

cystitis   Infection of the bladder.

dermatologist   Physician specializing in treating diseases of the skin.

discectomy   Surgical removal of a disc.

disease-modifying antirheumatic drugs (DMARDs)   Prescription medications used to treat rheumatoid and other inflammatory types of arthritis.

dystonia   Refers to the spasms felt in parts of the feet and the hands. For example, ankles or fingers may twist into uncomfortable positions; the feeling is one of cramping.

Eastern medicine   Refers to a variety of healing practices and products that originated in the Orient, from India to China and other countries in this area. Eastern medicine developed its own traditions. Its philosophy centers on restoring balance.

encephalitis   Inflammation of the brain.

endorphins   The body's "feel good" hormones. They're produced during periods of intense exercise and result in what's commonly known as the "runner's high."

endoscopy   Procedure in which a narrow flexible tube equipped with a light and a camera is inserted through a small incision or a natural opening, such as the nostril, to diagnose and allow repair of damaged tissue.

expectant management   Medical term for "watching and waiting."

fibromyalgia   Syndrome characterized by widespread pain, tender points, and fatigue.

fluoroscope   A medical imaging device that provides real-time images of the bony parts of the body. It uses an x-ray source and a display screen. The x-rays pass through the individual and are displayed on the screen.

fluoroscopy   Procedure that uses x-rays to observe the body's internal organs in real time.

gallstone   A solid crystal deposit, usually made up of cholesterol. Gallstones can range from the size of a grain of sand to the size of a golf ball.

gastroenterologist   Physician who specializes in diagnosing and treating disorders of the gastrointestinal tract. This tract includes the esophagus, stomach, small and large intestines, pancreas, liver, and gallbladder.

gout   Form of crystalline arthritis in which uric acid crystals build up in the joints.

hemophilia   Rare, genetically transmitted bleeding disorder.

hernia   Medical condition in which an internal organ protrudes through the muscle wall designed to hold it in place.

hinge joint   Gets its name because it opens and closes just like a door hinge. The knee is one of the body's biggest and heaviest hinge joints. It's also capable of slight rotating and twisting movements.

human genome project   Scientific endeavor completed in 2003 that resulted in sequencing and mapping every gene in the human body.

human papilloma virus (HPV)   Sexually transmitted virus linked to genital warts and cervical cancer.

iliac crest   The rim of the ilium, the big bone located at the upper portion of the pelvis. You can feel the iliac crest with your hands when you press in along your sides just below the waist.

invasive procedure   Term used to describe any medical procedure that cuts through or enters the skin. It also refers to the insertion of any medical devices into the body. An injection is a minimally invasive procedure.

lactic acid   Produced in your muscles during strenuous exercise, as blood sugar (glucose) is metabolized.

laminectomy   Surgical removal of the lamina, the posterior arch of a vertebra.

laparoscopic surgery   Modern minimally invasive surgical technique that uses a laparascope, a medical device guided by a camera and computer technology.

leptin   Hormone that plays an important role in metabolizing fat.

lower GI series   Diagnostic test that examines the lower intestine.

lupus   *See* systemic lupus erythematosus (SLE).

metatarsal bones   The long bones in your foot that extend from your ankle to the bases of your toes.

nerve block   Injection of anesthetic near a nerve to provide temporary pain relief.

neurologist   Physician who treats disorders of the nervous system.

neuropathies   Nerve disorders common in people with diabetes. Anywhere from 60 to 70 percent of diabetics will have nerve damage that can range from irritating to extremely painful.

nonsteroidal anti-inflammatory drugs (NSAIDs)   Class of medications used to reduce inflammation and relieve pain.

nuclear radiology   Field of radiology that uses radioactive material to send signals that can be recorded by a camera scanner.

orthotics   Devices designed to support various body structures or to correct musculoskeletal deformities.

osteochondromatosis   Rare medical condition in which cartilage-covered bony growths proliferate on a bone surface.

osteomalacia   Softening of the bones. Often referred to as rickets.

osteomyelitis   Bone infection usually caused by a bacterium.

otoscope   Handheld device with a light and a funnel-shaped attachment at one end. The attachment fits into the external ear canal, and the light allows a doctor to see inside the ear.

Paget's disease   Chronic bone condition in which bones become enlarged and misshapen.

pancreatitis   Inflammation of the pancreas.

peritonitis   Inflammation of the lining of the abdominal wall.

pheochromocytoma   Tumor of the adrenal gland.

phototherapy   Also called light therapy. Uses natural or ultraviolet light to treat symptoms generally associated with psoriasis or other conditions.

physiatrist   Physical medicine and rehabilitation physician, otherwise known as a "PMR" physician. Also treats disorders of the neuromuscular system.

placebo   A harmless substance that holds no medical benefit. It's used to evaluate the effects of a treatment in a comparison study.

polycythemia vera   Rare blood disorder in which the bone marrow overproduces red blood cells.

postherpetic neuralgia   Caused by the activation in adults of the dormant varicella-zoster virus that caused chickenpox.

prostaglandins   Found throughout the body, they're hormonelike entities and are responsible for many different body functions.

psychotherapist   Someone with a Master's or a doctorate in one of the mental health disciplines who provides counseling and therapy. Psychotherapists can be psychiatrists, registered psychiatric nurses, licensed counselors, or clinical social workers.

pyelonephritis   Infection of the kidneys.

referred pain   Occurs when you feel pain in one part of your body but the source is somewhere else. For example, pain associated with a heart attack may be felt in the left arm. This condition occurs because different nerve impulses are traveling along the same nerve pathway.

Reye's syndrome   In children and adolescents, a potentially life-threatening complication of aspirin use.

rheumatic fever   Inflammatory disease that may develop after a streptococcal infection.

sciatica   Painful condition caused by inflammation of the sciatic nerve.

shingles   *See* postherpetic neuralgia.

sickle cell anemia   Genetically transmitted blood disease.

skin biopsy   Procedure in which a doctor takes a small sample of skin tissue and then sends it to a lab for analysis.

spinal stenosis   A painful condition resulting from the narrowing of the space between discs in the spine.

staph   Shortened term for staphylococcus, commonly occurring bacterium that can cause infection.

steroids   Synthetic drugs given orally or as an injection to treat a variety of inflammatory medical conditions.

stimulus   Anything that produces a response.

strep   Shortened form of streptococcus, commonly occurring bacterium that can cause infection.

stressor   Any kind of stimulus that activates your body's stress response. It can be short term or chronic.

systemic lupus erythematosus (SLE)   Chronic inflammatory autoimmune disease affecting the joints as well as various internal organs.

temporomandibular joint disorder   Also known as TMJ, painful condition involving the jaw, jaw joint, and muscles in the surrounding area.

trigger finger   Painful condition of the hand in which the tendon of one or more fingers becomes inflamed and cannot easily fit through the tendon sheath.

triage   Process by which patients are sorted according to the severity of their medical conditions and need for medical care.

upper GI series   Diagnostic test of the upper intestine.

urethritis   Infection of the urethra.

X-STOP   Stands for Interspinous Process Decompression System. The device was approved by the FDA in 2005.

Alliance of State Pain Initiatives
University of Wisconsin
School of Medicine and Public Health
Room 4720
1300 University Avenue
Madison, WI 53706
aspi@mailplus.wisc.edu
http://aspi.wisc.edu/index.htm

The Alliance of State Pain Initiatives (ASPI) is a national network of interdisciplinary, state-based organizations dedicated to transforming the culture of pain care. ASPI, which is a program of the Carbone Comprehensive Cancer Center at the University of Wisconsin School of Medicine and Public Health, develops educational, advocacy, and quality improvement programs and provides resources and guidance to the State Pain Initiatives.

The ALS Association, National Office
27001 Agoura Road, Suite 250
Calabasas Hills, CA 91301-5104
Phone: 818-880-9007
Fax: 818-880-9006
www.alsa.org

The ALS Association is committed to leading the fight to cure and treat amyotrophic lateral sclerosis, also known as Lou Gehrig's Disease, through global, cutting-edge research, and to empower people with ALS and their families to live fuller lives by providing them with compassionate care and support.

American Academy of Orthopaedic Surgeons
6300 North River Road
Rosemont, IL 60018-4262
1-800-346-2267
www.aaos.org

Information on orthopaedic conditions and treatments, injury prevention, wellness and exercise, and more.

American Academy of Pain Management
www.aapainmanage.org

The American Academy of Pain Management (the Academy) is a nonprofit organization that educates clinicians about pain and its management through an integrative interdisciplinary approach. The Academy provides an environment for clinicians from a variety of health-care disciplines to network and share knowledge for optimal patient care.

The American Academy of Pain Medicine
4700 W. Lake Avenue
Glenview, IL 60025
847-375-4731
info@painmed.org
www.painmed.org

The American Academy of Pain Medicine (AAPM) is the medical specialty society representing physicians practicing in the field of pain medicine. As a medical specialty society, the Academy is involved in education, training, advocacy, and research in the specialty of pain medicine.

American Cancer Society
1-800-ACS-2345
www.cancer.org

The American Cancer Society (ACS) is a nationwide, community-based voluntary health organization. Headquartered in Atlanta, Georgia, the ACS has state divisions and more than 3,400 local offices.

American College of Rheumatology
1800 Century Place, Suite 250
Atlanta, GA 30345-4300
www.rheumatology.org

An organization of and for physicians, health professionals, and scientists that advances rheumatology through programs of education, research, advocacy, and practice support that foster excellence in the care of people with arthritis and rheumatic and musculoskeletal diseases.

American Council for Headache Education
19 Mantua Road
Mount Royal, NJ 08061
856-423-0043, Option 1
www.achenet.org

ACHE is an acronym for the American Headache Society (AHS) Council for Headache Education. ACHE is sponsored and directed by AHS, which is a professional society of health-care providers dedicated to the study and treatment of headache and face pain. Founded in 1959, AHS brings together physicians and other health providers from various fields and specialties to share concepts and developments about headache and related conditions.

American Diabetes Association
AskADA@diabetes.org.
www.diabetes.org

The American Diabetes Association is leading the fight against the deadly consequences of diabetes and fighting for those affected by diabetes. The Association funds research to prevent, cure, and manage diabetes; delivers services to hundreds of communities; provides objective and credible information; and gives voice to those denied their rights because of diabetes.

American Heart Association
National Center
7272 Greenville Avenue
Dallas, TX 75231
1-800-242-8721
www.americanheart.org

Provides education, information, and lifestyle tips for living with and preventing coronary artery disease.

American Pain Foundation
201 North Charles Street, Suite 710
Baltimore, MD 21201-4111
http://action.painfoundation.org

The American Pain Foundation is an independent nonprofit organization serving people with pain through information, advocacy, and support. Their mission is to improve the quality of life of people with pain by raising public awareness, providing practical information, promoting research, and advocating to remove barriers and increase access to effective pain management.

American Pain Society
4700 W. Lake Avenue
Glenview, IL 60025
847-375-4715
info@ampainsoc.org
www.ampainsoc.org

The American Pain Society is a multidisciplinary community that brings together a diverse group of scientists, clinicians, and other professionals to increase the knowledge of pain and transform public policy and clinical practice to reduce pain-related suffering.

American Thyroid Association
www.thyroid.org

The American Thyroid Association (ATA) is the leading organization focused on thyroid biology and the prevention and treatment of thyroid disorders through excellence and innovation in research, clinical care, education, and public health.

Arthritis Foundation
PO Box 7669
Atlanta, GA 30357-0669
1-800-283-7800
www.arthritis.org

The Arthritis Foundation is the only national not-for-profit organization that supports the more than 100 types of arthritis and related conditions. The Arthritis Foundation offers information and tools to help people live a better life with arthritis.

HIV/AIDS
www.aids.gov
www.nlm.nih.gov/medlineplus/aids.html

The first web address is the U.S. government website dedicated to providing resources on HIV/AIDS. The second is a service of the U.S. National Library of Medicine and the National Institutes of Health.

National Center for Complementary and Alternative Medicine
9000 Rockville Pike
Bethesda, MD 20892
info@nccam.nih.gov
nccam.nih.gov

The federal government's lead agency for scientific research on complementary and alternative medicine (CAM) and 1 of the 27 institutes and centers that make up the National Institutes of Health within the U.S. Department of Health and Human Services.

National Fibromyalgia Association
2121 S. Towne Centre Place, Suite 300
Anaheim, CA 92806
714-921-0150
www.fmaware.org

The National Fibromyalgia Association is a nonprofit organization whose mission is to develop and execute programs dedicated to improving the quality of life for people with fibromyalgia.

The National Foundation for the Treatment of Pain
1714 White Oak Drive
Houston, TX 77009
713-862-9332
www.paincare.org

The National Foundation for the Treatment of Pain is a not-for-profit organization dedicated to providing support for patients who are suffering from intractable pain. The Foundation also provides support to their families, friends, and the physicians who treat them.

National Headache Foundation
820 N. Orleans, Suite 217
Chicago, IL 60610
info@headaches.org
www.headaches.org

The National Headache Foundation (NHF) provides educational and informational resources, supporting headache research and advocating for the understanding of headache as a legitimate neurobiological disease.

National Institute of Arthritis and Musculoskeletal and Skin Diseases
1 AMS Circle
Bethesda, MD 20892-3675
1-877-22N-IAMS (226-4267)
TTY: 301-565-2966
niamsinfo@mail.nih.gov
www.niams.nih.gob

Supports research into the causes, treatment, and prevention of arthritis and musculoskeletal and skin diseases, the training of basic and clinical scientists to carry out this research, and the dissemination of information on research progress in these diseases.

National Institute of Neurological Disorders and Stroke
www.ninds.nih.gov/disorders/reflex_sympathetic_dystrophy/
reflex_sympathetic_dystrophy.htm

Information on Complex Regional Pain Syndrome from the National Institutes of Health.

National Institutes of Health
9000 Rockville Pike
Bethesda, MD 20892
www.nih.gov

The National Institutes of Health (NIH) is part of the U.S. Department of Health and Human Services and the primary federal agency for conducting and supporting medical research.

The National Migraine Association/M.A.G.N.U.M.
100 North Union Street, Suite B
Alexandria, VA 22314
www.migraines.org

Created to bring public awareness, utilizing the electronic, print, and artistic mediums, to the fact that Migraine is a true biologic neurological disease; to assist Migraine sufferers, their families, and coworkers; and to help improve the quality of life of Migraine sufferers worldwide. (M.A.G.N.U.M. stands for **M**igraine **A**wareness **G**roup: A **N**ational **U**nderstanding for **M**igraineurs.)

National Multiple Sclerosis Society
1-800-344-4867
www.nationalmssociety.org

The Society helps people affected by multiple sclerosis (MS) by funding cutting-edge research, driving change through advocacy, facilitating professional education, and providing programs and services that help people with MS and their families move their lives forward.

The National Spinal Cord Injury Association (NSCIA)
1-800-962-9629
www.spinalcord.org

Dedicated to educate and empower survivors of spinal cord injury and disease to achieve and maintain the highest levels of independence, health, and personal fulfillment.

National Stroke Association
www.stroke.org

Information on stroke risk factors, symptoms, prevention, and recovery.

Pain & the Law
www.painandthelaw.org

Information on legal issues, advocacy, and current research on pain.

PainPathways: **Official Magazine of the World Institute of Pain**
www.painpathways.org

Quarterly magazine for acute, chronic, and cancer pain management.

Parkinson's Disease Foundation
1359 Broadway, Suite 1509
New York, NY 10018
212-923-4700
www.pdf.org

The Parkinson's Disease Foundation (PDF) is a leading national presence in Parkinson's disease research, education, and public advocacy.

Shingles (Herpes Zoster)
www.nlm.nih.gov/medlineplus/ency/article/000858.htm

Information from the National Institutes of Health on Shingles.

Index